ORAL HISTORY
FOR THE QUALITATIVE RESEARCHER

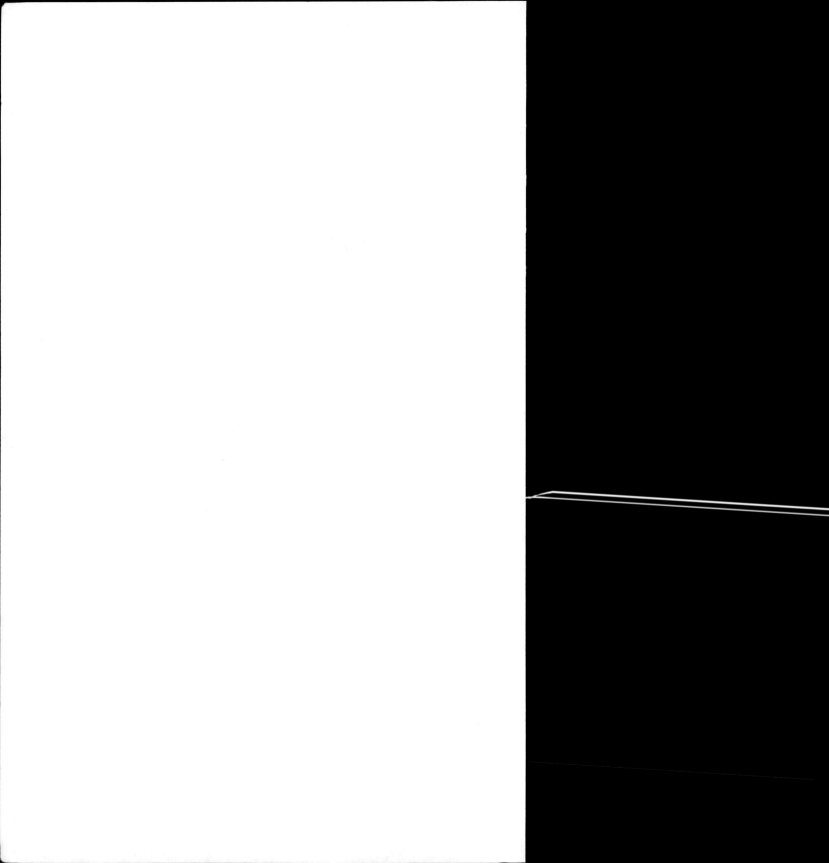

ORAL HISTORY
FOR THE QUALITATIVE
RESEARCHER

Choreographing the Story

Valerie J. Janesick

THE GUILFORD PRESS
New York   London

Library of Congress Cataloging-in-Publication Data
Janesick, Valerie J.
  Oral history for the qualitative researcher : choreographing the story /
Valerie J. Janesick.
    p. cm.
  Includes bibliographical references and index.
  ISBN 978-1-59385-073-9 (pbk.: alk. paper) — ISBN 978-1-60623-556-0
(hardcover: alk. paper)
  1. Oral history.   2. Qualitative research.   I. Title.
  D16.14.J36 2010
  001.4′33—dc22
                                                             2009046569

PREFACE

I have often said that I did not find oral history; rather, oral history found me. I have been fortunate throughout my career to work with advanced graduate students, many of them in the fields of education and the social sciences, and I was struck by the situation in which they found themselves. They were articulate, critically adept, and powerful writers. They were earning doctorates in education or the social sciences. They were sophisticated and excellent teachers in their respective settings. By virtue of earning a doctorate, they would leave their pre-K–12 classrooms to move on in their careers. Ironically, I was inadvertently somewhat responsible for helping talented teachers leave the classroom. I was prompted to give them one instruction for their oral histories: Describe yourself and your work as you move to your new position in the workforce. They were at a major transition point in their lives, and that is always a good time for an oral history interview. Little did I know what would follow, as is the case with qualitative interviews in general. In effect, each time I gave this instruction I realized that I had to document a fascinating set of cases, an oral history project of people who leave or move on in their current professions but who transform the essence of teaching into a new career. In this book, you will see examples of testimony from several members of this project—the very project that got me involved in articulating the methodology of oral history for qualitative researchers. It also inspired me to propose an oral history study of female school superintendents for a small in-house (University of South Florida) College of Education mini-grant in 2007–2008. You will see some sections of those oral histories in this book as well.*

Throughout my own career as a qualitative researcher, I have constantly sought ways to refine our methods and to emphasize methodological rigor. I thought about reinventing oral history, by which I mean that it may be time to go beyond the documentary techniques and think of new ways to represent interview transcripts and archival data and documents. For me, poetry-, photography-, and arts-based approaches to representation work well and are described in the book. Most other oral history books on the market (or even free on the Web) deal with the "how-to" aspect of oral history (e.g., Frisch, 1990; Hoopes, 1979; Perks & Thomson, 2006; Ritchie, 2003; Yow, 1994, 2005). A major goal of this book is to go beyond this excellent groundwork to open up our repertoire of techniques, much like the modern dance choreographers did for the dance repertoire in going beyond the classical ballets. Unfortunately, qualitative research in general and oral history in particular have been assaulted on a regular basis, as if they were not worthy of being called research. This is a sad indictment of our times and of the shortsightedness of some critics. Thus I wanted to write a book to explain and widen the repertoire of techniques available to researchers interested in documenting the lives of ordinary people through oral history. I add elements of testimony as oral history, oral history as a social justice project, photovoice, constructing poetry from interview data as found data poems, and digital oral history.

In a sense, you may also think of this book as emergent oral history, part of a growing body of literature on emergent qualitative methods (see Frisch, 2008; Hesse-Biber & Leavy, 2008). Because qualitative work and oral history often include the voices and stories of those on the margins of society, I hope this book contributes to some awareness of social justice. Because women have been excluded from oral history projects on a regular basis in the past century, obviously the feminist research methods texts offer us some understanding of feminist oral history (Hesse-Biber & Leavy, 2007;

---

* Transcripts have been edited to allow for clear readability.

Reinharz, 1992). Wherever possible, I add Web resources, as the Internet is exploding with oral history projects, particularly on You-Tube, MySpace, Second Life, and Facebook. I also include relevant blogs, which are rich resources for all qualitative researchers, especially oral historians. One only has to look at YouTube or Facebook to see the constant updating and recording of someone's life. For oral historians, going digital can only assist in illuminating the powerful stories people tell us about their lived experience.

I believe my interest in oral history comes from a deep appreciation of history and a love of qualitative research methods as a way to understand society, the self, and my own autobiography. Early in my own life, I was taken with reading history, autobiography, biography, and the classics. Concurrently, I was studying dance and choreography, which grew to be my reference point for making sense of storytelling, not just through dance but through my work as a researcher. This led me to other classic historical and artistic texts by Barbara Tuchman, Paul Thompson, Valerie Yow, and others. I was also greatly influenced by Studs Terkel (1912–2008), the oral history icon and one of the great writers of our times. I noticed that the work of the historian and artist parallels that of the qualitative researcher, and vice versa.

From my theoretical stance of critical pedagogy and the writings of John Dewey, Paulo Freire, Henry Giroux, Joe Kincheloe, Shirley Steinberg, and Donaldo Macedo, I also view oral history as a positive way to advance social justice. Most recently, the work in memory and narrative by Mary Chamberlain and Paul Thompson and Carolyn Ellis's work on researching subjectivity have had a deep impact on my thinking. Finally, the work on digital history and Internet inquiry were welcome pieces in the puzzle of making sense of oral history in the technological/digital era.

Having experienced and survived the trauma of four hurricanes in 2004, I took an introspective turn and decided to get all my research notes and transcripts together and put my thoughts down on paper. The result is *Oral History for the Qualitative Researcher: Choreographing the Story*.

As a former choreographer, I have used the metaphor of dance and the arts in earlier works (Janesick, 2000, 2004) and continue to use the metaphor in this book. I am transferring what I know of choreography to illuminate our understanding of oral history. The metaphor is extended here to help those who wish to learn more about oral history as a tool for qualitative researchers.

This book is not a detailed step-by-step methods guide. I describe technique as needed, but, in thinking like a choreographer and a historian, I try to evoke an understanding of potential ways to make sense of an oral history project after the transcripts. You will see descriptions of interview technique, of journal writing as a research technique, and of archival research and the use of photography and video techniques—all of which are heuristic tools or guides for qualitative researchers who want to know more about oral history as a technique and as a path to social justice, as well as for those new to oral history who want to learn about multiple approaches to doing oral history.

This book is intended for beginner, intermediate, and practicing researchers and those in training. No matter at what level the reader finds him- or herself, I ask that all who read this text read with *the eye of the beginner*, which allows for an open, even awestruck, awareness at times of any and all age-old topics. I use the terms *order*, *design*, *tension*, *balance and composition*, and *harmony*, as they are critical elements in dance and choreography and fit well with the oral historian's work. Part I of the book deals with the connections between oral history, qualitative research, and the principles of choreography (*order*). Part II is about techniques of oral history (*design and tension*); ethical, legal, and institutional review board issues; and the relevance of oral history for our times. Parts III and IV discuss meaning, interpretation, using poetry and visual data, and action (*balance and composition*, and *harmony*). These parts discuss the role of the qualitative researcher as oral historian, testimony as oral history, and oral history as a social justice project.

Throughout, I integrate examples of oral history interviews with examples of the researcher's reflective journal entries on the given project. At the request of some participants in my oral history projects and to ensure whatever modicum of privacy is left in our information age, I have changed the actual names of places and participants and have used last names of great and favorite choreographers to capture the essence of participants. Wherever possible, I integrate commentary and examples of social justice implications in oral history work.

I also chose to write in user-friendly language and not in the academic writing genre to make this work accessible to a larger population—those who do oral history as independent work for communities and libraries, for example.

Certain tragic events in our social history, such as the debacle of Hurricane Katrina, made the world aware of major disparities in our society, of personal heartbreaking tragedies, of all that is troublesome about bureaucratic inefficiency and corruption, of how we are connected as individuals, and of the importance of oral history as a social justice project. In fact, many oral histories of survivors of the hurricane have been and are being recorded on film, such as Spike Lee's documentary *When the Levees Broke: A Requiem in Four Acts.*

I dedicate this book to those who perished as a result of Hurricane Katrina, to the survivors, to the workers who continue to assist these individuals, and to all my students, colleagues, and reviewers. The death in 2008 of Studs Terkel, the oral historian who inspired me, compels me to dedicate this book to him as well.

VALERIE J. JANESICK

ACKNOWLEDGMENTS

There are many people whose names do not appear on the cover whom I wish to thank for their assistance in writing this book. For illustrative purposes, I relied on many examples from individuals whose names have been changed. However, I wish to express my gratitude to them personally: Lorna Elam, Carolyn N. Stevenson, Alonzo Westbrook, Judy Castillo, Craig Collins, Patricia Williams Boyd, Terry Bigelow, Kristy Loman Chiodo, and Jan Mulqueeny. These current and former students have already distinguished themselves as able researchers, historians, and writers, and I am grateful for their presence in my life. In addition, my gratitude and affection go to my editor, C. Deborah Laughton, who is the essence of patience as well as a true friend and spirit guide. Many thanks as well to the entire team of reviewers for their help and guidance: William G. Tierney, University of Southern California; Brad Schultz, Northeastern Illinois University; and Patrick M. Jenlink, Stephen F. Austin State University. I thank the editorial team at The Guilford Press, especially MaryBeth Woods, Paul Gordon, Anna Nelson, and the many others involved in marketing, production, graphics, and design for the book. Finally, I thank all my doctoral students who love oral history and qualitative research narrative work. They always raised the perfect questions to challenge my thinking. I appreciate their enthusiasm, generosity, and overall goodness. As a result, I have great faith in the next generation of researchers.

CONTENTS

PART IV. HARMONY   179
The Art of Making Sense of Oral History Projects with a Choreography of Social Justice

ORAL HISTORY
FOR THE QUALITATIVE RESEARCHER

PART I

~

ORDER

Reinventing Oral History
for the Qualitative Researcher

We tell ourselves stories in order to live.
—JOAN DIDION

INTRODUCTION

The power of oral history lies in the power of storytelling. Whether an oral history project embraces and describes the story of one person's life or a collection of individual stories told together, the power resides in the meaning made of the storytelling and what we learn from the stories. Although there are quite a few books on oral history methods, in this book I focus on oral history for the qualitative researcher, with an emphasis on oral history as a social justice project and how using poetry may augment representation of oral history data. Because oral history captures the lived experience of a person or persons, the social justice goals become more definite when the stories are of those left on the periphery of society. Oral history is a vehicle for the outsiders and the forgotten to tell their stories. In recent history, the many sets of oral histories of the 9/11 Oral History Project are just one example of how oral history can be used

1

to help understand current events through the lived experience of participants. Another fine example is Steven Spielberg's Survivors of the Shoah Visual History Archive housed at the University of Southern California Shoah Foundation Institute. In the Shoah (Holocaust) study, oral histories document events of World War II through the words of the survivors and their families. Both of these examples are discussed further later in this book. In addition, the oral history project of Hurricane Katrina survivors serves to punctuate the underlying social justice implications of doing oral history. I use the metaphor of choreography as needed to illustrate key points, as choreography is all about telling a story through dance. In oral history we tell the story through spoken text, written text, video text, or all of these media.

Oral history is a technique with its very own history (see Thompson, 1988). Oral history grew out of the oral tradition. Formal written work about oral history emerged in the last century. Since then we have experienced many evolutionary stages in the development of the field. Today we are in the center of a monumental stage—the digital movement. Digital technology enables us to move forward, experimenting with new lenses and technologies. This leads us to ask, What is oral history? There are many definitions of oral history, but for this book, I define oral history as it is often understood in this era:

> *Oral history is the collection of stories and reminiscences of a person or persons who have firsthand knowledge of any number of experiences.*

Naturally, because oral history projects span multiple disciplines in addition to history, there are multiple approaches and multiple types of oral history. For example, you may find in the literature **standalone individual oral histories**. This type of oral history relies on one person's story, often in a type of stream-of-consciousness narrative, may be analyzed or not, and may be in tape format or printed as hard text. Another type of oral history is a **collective oral history**. Here you may find many individual stories around a particular theme or stories in which all people share a particular experience. For example, the current oral histories being taped of Hurricane

Katrina survivors, when published, would constitute a collective of many individual stories similar to the 9/11 oral history and memory project. Another collection or set of oral histories might include those kept by the U.S. military. The military has an extensive collection of oral histories, and, in fact, their guide to doing oral history is on the World Wide Web. The collection of oral histories includes the testimonials of soldiers returning from war; currently, these include the soldiers returning from Iraq. Sometimes a collection of oral histories may follow a theme, such as Steven Spielberg's Survivors of the Shoah project. On the other hand, stand-alone oral histories of the individual genre may also rely on themes but take an idiosyncratic approach. To offer a few examples, the University of South Florida (USF) is in the process of collecting oral histories through various projects, such as:

1. Oral histories of prominent individuals in the field of public health, collected to better understand the field from their perspectives.

2. The USF 25th and 50th Anniversary Projects, collecting information from faculty, staff, students, and alumni.

3. West Central Florida Land Use Project.

4. Florida Citrus Industry Project on the impact of globalization on the industry.

5. The *Tampa Tribune* Project, collecting oral histories from staff writers of this newspaper.

In addition, at least a dozen local oral history projects are under way here in Tampa alone. Regardless of the type of oral history, oral historians rely on intensive interviewing of one genre or another, such as the long interview. Many oral historians—myself included—prefer to interview a participant over time, more than once and as needed to get a fuller picture and more detail. This type of interviewing relies on what Rubin and Rubin (2005) call **hearing** the data, or qualitative interviewing. Clark (1999) also reminds us that oral history is "located in the space between ethnography, sociology, and history" (p. 3), mostly qualitative disciplines. The connection for me to dance is natural. In dance, the choreographer and dancer together tell a story through the performance of the dance, just as the oral historian eventually must tell the story of the participants in the study. In the postmodern era, this story can be any person's story. This is the social justice link. Instead of interviewing only prominent or elite participants, now all voices have the potential to be documented. With ease, this can be facilitated by access to media such as photographs, videos, blogs, vlogs (video logs), and social networking sites.

Early in the last century, oral history focused on interviewing elite persons, such as generals, famous artists or scientists, great leaders of nations, and anyone who surfaced as distinctive. At the same time, local individuals who had a strong memory of a town, city, state, or region were sometimes seen as knowledgeable only in terms of historical events, not necessarily in terms of their own lived experience of those events. Thus it is helpful to view oral history itself on a continuum in order to understand where we are in this time period. On one end, the most sophisticated individual elite may be interviewed; on the other end, we have the most ordinary everyday citizen. Each person has much to tell us as we come to understand society in all its complexity.

Of course, the specific techniques of oral history are also the techniques of the qualitative researcher—the techniques of interview, observation, document analysis, journal writing, and, more recently, digital photography and videotaping and analysis. Likewise, the use of ordinary language to convey a story has its roots in qualitative research. It is easy to see how oral history can be a valuable tool in the qualitative researcher's tool kit, so to speak. Furthermore, we as qualitative researchers have experienced various transformations, from a traditionalist to a reconceptualist approach and now to the postmodern orientation. Consequently, I argue in this text that oral history can be extended to be understood as a postmodern social justice project by virtue of including those voices of individuals left on the margins and periphery of society or those generally forgotten. Many such stories will raise questions for our society from the oral histories that are documented. In my own field of education, I hope that oral history will be considered as a solid and viable approach to research for dissertations. In the field of education, although qualitative work in general and narrative approaches such as oral history are gaining acceptability, respectability, and use, we still have a long way to go. The reasons are the long tradition of quantitative research approaches used in education and the deep-seated influence of educational psychology in our work. Practically speaking, as grant money evaporates for work in the social sciences, oral history becomes a manageable approach to research for full-time working students, as the cost of travel and transcriptions is far less than the cost of using other approaches to research.

ORAL HISTORY EVOLVING AND A WORK IN PROGRESS

In this book, I take a dynamic view of oral history. I am asking the reader to give up the notion that oral history is simply a collection of tapes and transcripts on file in a library archive. There are many oral histories sitting on library shelves, and that is where they stay; they may never have been checked out or listened to. Rather, I am asking the reader to take a journey with me in viewing oral history as dynamic, ever changing, and evolving to match the evolution in our understanding of research and society.

Any research project requires analysis and interpretation. In the postmodern era, oral history can indeed consist of tapes and transcripts and other documents. However, that is only the first step. In the next step, analysis and interpretation, how we represent our data becomes important. For example, in my case, I try to use poetry to capture the themes of a given oral history project through found data poems, that is, poems constructed from the words of the narrator of the oral history. Then the question becomes, What can we learn from oral histories? Thus the interviewer as oral historian shares an interpretive role with the participant being interviewed. This in turn may become part of raising social justice questions. In fact, in my own collective oral history research project on women teachers, a participant asked me, "What are you calling me in the write-up?" I answered that I usually use the word "participant" to describe members in a study. She then said to me, "Wouldn't it be better to call us both interpreters?" She then went on to say that she gave so much thought to the interview questions and her responses that she, in fact, could not stop thinking about her role as a middle school teacher turned professor of teacher education. What she was talking about was the evolutionary, vibrant nature of oral history. Thus for me the reason for connecting oral history to this moment in time with qualitative research rests on the notion of interpretation.

Why do we want to hear the stories of individuals? Why do we take pains to record on tape and even type transcripts of stories about the past? Why do researchers undertake such projects? We do this to understand the lives of those whom we interview in order to understand ourselves and our worlds. Thus oral history becomes particularly useful to qualitative researchers, for we are regularly documenting multiple histories of multiple individuals to make sense of our world. Experience and what sense we make of experience are critical components of our work. Here is where oral history and qualitative research meet. We converge in various ways:

1. The *basic techniques* of oral history are the basic techniques of qualitative research. Both use interviews, observations, documents, photographs, videos, and drawings as evidence.

2. The researcher is the research instrument in oral history, as in qualitative research approaches in general. Just as the dancer stretches to sharpen technique, the oral historian sharpens and stretches the research instrument, too. Sharpening listening skills to hear the data is one part of the equation. Then sharpening the eyes to observe and really see the context of the narrator/interviewee is another. Practicing narrative writing and sharpening and exercising the fingers as one writes in coordination with the brain is yet another. When one is aware that the body is the research instrument in this type of work, the eventual narrative product is more focused, sharper, and nuanced. This comes with practice.

3. Telling someone's story, particularly through remembering key events and *lived experience,* is a major goal both for the oral historian and for many qualitative research projects.

4. Using *ordinary language* to tell the story is required for both the oral historian and the qualitative researcher.

5. There is *no one set explanation or interpretation for a given set of data.* Oral historians as qualitative researchers use the data at

hand and render the best explanation and interpretation possible at that moment in time.

6. Historians and qualitative researchers in general are involved in *describing and explaining someone's recollection* of events and activities. It is a memory of the self.

7. *Oral historians and qualitative researchers, like the choreographer, fashion a narrative to represent the lived experience,* and analysis and interpretation by the researcher and participant are often left open to further interpretation by the audience for the narrative. In other words, all good narratives have a point of view, and any audience may agree or disagree with the narrative. Readers of an oral history are like audience members experiencing a dance concert.

8. Oral historians include the voices of all potential participants, thereby acknowledging *multiculturalism* and *diversity* by documenting the stories of women, minorities, the disabled, and *those generally excluded from research* in general.

9. Oral history and qualitative research work in general validate a public pedagogy. That is, the documentation of someone's lived experience invites public reading, dialogue, and discussion. A person's lived experience is impossible to invalidate.

10. Oral history and qualitative work in general resist collapsing into some market entity. At least up to this point, no marketers have taken to oral history, and it has not been appropriated for mass marketing and ownership. In other words, oral history is not chasing money; it cannot be consumed and cannot be resold as some marketable product. It is what it is.

11. Oral history and qualitative research projects in general may raise uncomfortable and troublesome social questions that may ultimately affect social policy. For example, the number of firsthand accounts of 9/11 and those of Hurricane Katrina survivors may to some extent have influenced subsequent social policy on homeland security, for example, and the Environmental Protection Agency.

Likewise, consider that oral history has been around for all of time. In whatever era humankind has developed and evolved, real stories of persons' lives have been told. Consider the following time line as you process the connection between oral history techniques and qualitative research techniques. I use this as a broad overview for students starting an oral history project.

Traditionalist era	Reconceptualist era	Postmodernist era
• Cave paintings to taped recordings • Storytelling as basic component told from generation to generation	• Taped recordings on audiotape and videotape • Writing • Storytelling continues; may be tied to a social issue and use of analysis for change	• Taped interview • Observations • Co-researching • Digital stories • Storytelling is co-constructed and possibly ties to a social issue with additional analysis and awareness of social justice

Oral History in Traditionalist Era

- Marked by social circumstances of the time; tells someone's story with tools at hand (e.g., cave painting, hieroglyphs, petroglyphs, oral tradition).

- Developed in the technological age into recordings on tape and some photography, usually documenting the remembered history of well-known elites, such as generals, corporate leaders, and famous citizens.

- Storyteller primarily constructs the narrative.

- Researcher takes special care to avoid interpretation.

- Stories usually of great male warriors or leaders.

- Stories primarily told of those in power.

- Often, even in the last century, consisted of taped interviews stored in a library or archive to be checked out for listening.

Oral History in Reconceptualist Era

- Uses audiotapes and possibly videotapes, photography, and interactive interviews; beginning of naming interviewers and interviewees as co-researchers; sometimes cowriting the text as well.

- Beginning to identify a theoretical frame for analysis of interviews.

- Beginning to work with participants to craft the narrative.

- May have some social issue for the narrative.

- Validates the lived experience of the participants by member-checking information.

- Consists mostly of taped interviews on file in a library or archive.

- Beginning to note ethical issues and analysis of same, such as informed consent, confidentiality, anonymity.

Oral History of Postmodern Era

- Uses all possible audio, video, and written recording techniques.

- Includes participant in interpretation.

- Uses digital storytelling and co-researching.

- Co-constructs the narrative with participants.

- May tie the lived experience narrative purposefully to a social justice issue.

- May include newer theoretical frames for interpreting the narrative, such as feminist theories and critical theories.

- Acknowledges multiculturalism and diversity by documenting voices of those outside the mainstream of society.

- Resists marketers, marketing, and overall mass consumption.

- Purposely looks to document the stories of the outsiders in society, including women, minorities, disabled members, those who are not members of the mainstream group or society.

- Intentionally makes available on the Internet oral histories and oral history projects, in entirety, of a particular group, such as projects on YouTube.

- Includes ethical issues for discussion.
- Seeks transparency throughout the entire research project.

For the purpose of this book, I work predominately from a postmodern perspective to emphasize the evolution of oral history. In this perspective oral history takes on more texture and possibly more credibility. Thus *postmodern oral history* is characterized by:

- An interpretive approach that may include the participant in the project as a co-researcher.
- Both interviewer and interviewee taking active roles in the project.
- Use of ordinary language in the final report to make the story understandable to the widest possible audience.
- Use of technology to enhance the power of the story being told; may use multiple technologies and the written word to complete the storytelling; regular use of digital cameras, digital video cameras, cell phones, and other devices as part of the narrative itself; possible posting on YouTube or other Internet site for easier rapid access by a larger audience.
- Discussing ethical issues and bringing them to the forefront of the project and throughout the project.
- An approach to qualitative research work that continually persists and prevails in public spaces such as libraries and websites; one of the most transparent and most public of approaches, regardless of the discipline base, which may be history, sociology, education, gerontology, medicine, or others.
- A pride in validating the subjectivities of participants; acknowledging and celebrating subjectivity in order to reach new understanding of someone's lived experience.
- Inclusion of voices and stories of those members of society typically disenfranchised and marginalized for study and documentation.
- A view of oral history as a democratic project, acknowledging that any person's story may be documented using accessible

means to the data. For example, the New York City firefighters' oral history of 9/11 project (*www.freedomstories.org*) includes more than 12,000 pages of oral histories from 503 firefighters and emergency medical technicians. These oral histories are available on the Web (see Appendix A).

In addition, to use the metaphor of choreography to help in understanding oral history, it is helpful to understand something about the work of choreography. Not to oversimplify, but often the choreographer asks the following questions as a general beginning to any dance/art work. My favorite ballet teacher framed it this way:

Who (or what) is doing

What to whom (or what) and

Where, in what context, and

Why, what were the difficulties?

I wish to describe the ways in which choreography interfaces with oral history as a qualitative research technique, as I have done elsewhere (Janesick, 2000, 2004, 2007a). In oral history, eventually a finished report is completed. Completing this report is like choreographing a dance. The story or narrative of the dance is like the story or narrative of any given oral history. In dealing with the basic *who, what, where, why* of a story, it is inevitable that we get to the interpretation of someone's life as lived. Granted that a good deal of oral history work focuses on people experiencing traumatic events and stories of elites and quasi-elites, there is a steady movement, due to technology, toward documenting lives of ordinary people who have lived on the margins of society and who have stories to tell. All this is done while including a respect for history and for the memory of individuals and their lived experience. Memory is, in fact, often used as a synonym for the work of oral history. Sociologists, in particular, and others have written of the importance of memory, and oral historians value the memory of participants.

MNEMOSYNE, GODDESS OF MEMORY

It would be difficult to write about oral history without going back to Greek mythology for inspiration. In Greek storytelling Mnemosyne is the Titaness daughter of Gaia and Uranus who became the mother of the Muses by Zeus. Mnemosyne is considered pivotal in Greek mythology, for she is the goddess of and personification of memory. To be the holder of all memory was critical, for it was also Mnemosyne who discovered the power of thought, reason, and memory. She is said to have named every object, value, belief, and feeling on this earth. Because without language there would be little communication among mortals, she gave the power of memory and language to all mortals. The Greek story told of Mnemosyne is that Zeus visited her, and she bore the nine Muses, who are believed to have been born in this order:

Calliope, Muse of epic poetry

Clio, Muse of history

Nelpomene, Muse of tragedy

Enterpe, Muse of lyric poetry

Erato, Muse of love poetry

Terpsichore, Muse of dance and music

Urania, Muse of astronomy

Thàlia, Muse of comedy

Polymnia, Muse of sacred poetry

In Greek lore, the nine Muses preside over the arts and sciences and inspire us all. Obviously, historians and oral historians have an affinity for the symbolic importance of Clio, the Muse of history. In Web-based contemporary culture, there are numerous oral history projects named for Clio—for example, CLIOPATRIA, is a group blog, subtitled Oral History, at YouTube. Likewise, Mnemosyne is used in many digital stories as an avatar and as an action figure on so many sites on the World Wide Web that it would take days to visit them. In the classical world, poetics and the arts in general were thought to be a divine gift. If any mortal was an artist, that person was favored by the gods and goddesses. Poets, philosophers, and musicians were revered in Greek society as a result of this widely held notion. In addition, the thought patterns of the human psyche were believed to be manifested in the physical realm by the Muses and what they represented. The Muses were thought to ride the winged horse Pegasus to soar high above the earth to imagine and create poetry, music, dance, and so on. It is remarkable that in the evolution of medicine, to this day the center of the brain that houses memory is called the hippocampus. The word *hippocampus* means seahorse, which relates to Pegasus (whose father is Poseidon, god of the sea).

Thus the Greeks sought to explain the classical ideal of poetics as elevating the mortals in a kind of symmetry and beauty, something artists, especially choreographers, and some researchers do as well. Later writers such as Plato, Aristotle, Thucydides, Aristophanes, and others would extend theories and explanations of the human psyche and intellectual illumination with a nod to the goddess of memory, Mnemosyne. Poetry was important in Greek and subsequently Roman society. After all, Homer, in the *Iliad* and the *Odyssey*, recorded the stories of his society in the form of poetry, with an able storytelling narrator. One might think of history as a thread from the Greeks, running through Mnemosyne and Clio to the present day. So the question, Why oral history now? is of considerable and notable importance.

WHY ORAL HISTORY NOW?

Oral history is of interest in many disciplines—such as history, sociology, anthropology, nursing, mental health, medicine, education, and business—and to social science researchers in general. It may also be considered an art form employing the art of storytelling. Historical fiction based on firsthand oral and written historical accounts often provides powerful storytelling, such as the works of James Michener. His thoroughly researched works, such as *Hawaii*, *Texas*, *Chesapeake*, and others, were based on oral histories, documents, and his vivid imagination. Likewise, oral history is an interpretive activity of communication that is extremely active in the technological environment of the postmodern era. In addition, in this postmodern era, in-depth interviews are still the quintessential substantive dataset. Most important, memory is a fascinating part of the social world and of our individual lives and contributes to the documentation of oral history projects. When a person interviews another human being, the transcript becomes a written record. The knowledge of the past helps to refute myths, half-truths, fabrications, and faulty perspectives and validates the story of the lived experience being described.

In addition, with a renewed sense of interest in oral history, as evidenced by journal articles and books printed since the 1970s, there will always be an open space for qualitative researchers to pursue in-depth interviews in any given research project. Once a student asked me, "How do I know I am doing oral history?" As with any research project, the researcher has an idea of the history and foundations for designing a project and has some compelling need to find out about the lived experience of an individual or a group of individuals. There are a multitude of oral traditions, and one has to make a decision to learn about the tradition of choice, has to spell out clearly that tradition, and has to jump into doing the project. This is true of any type of research project, qualitative or quantitative. One would not, for example, simply send out a survey without being grounded in some theoretical perspective and knowledge of the processes of follow-up and statistical framework. Likewise, in any qualitative work a researcher needs to be able to identify, describe, and explain the perspective of an oral history project, as well as the compelling nature of the inquiry. Because this book is about oral history as a qualitative *research* technique, that is what I focus on; it is not my intent to differentiate it from every possible other qualitative technique, such as ethnography, case studies, action research, or other field-based studies.

SORTING OUT ORAL TRADITIONS

Some writers seem to feel that there is only one way to define oral history. The reason may be various terms are used interchangeably.

Some of the terms include *oral history, folklore, memory, déjà-vu, narrative, storytelling, autobiography, autoethnography, portraiture, biography,* the *long interview, reminiscence, photovoice, life history,* and *photoethnography.* I list these terms not to confuse the issue but to point out that each of these terms overlap in many ways. For example, they overlap in their overall **purpose**—that is, to tell someone's story. They overlap in **method**—that is, using interviews and some written documents as primary research techniques. They overlap in **rationale** in terms of the need to uncover stories from the past so that we can preserve more than a bureaucratic account of a person's life. A bureaucratic account might consist of a person's social security number, driver's license, business cards, deeds of sale, bank account records, and will. True, these can give some fascinating information regarding a person's life, and an oral historian may include them to complement a life story. But in the oral history genre, we seek to get the real texture of the story of a real person's life in all its depth, complexity, misery, joy, and purpose. By telling a real person's story we create a **sense of history**, and this can accomplish much:

1. A sense of history empowers us.
2. A sense of history may serve to illuminate the present situation.
3. A sense of history forces us to make sense of who we are.
4. A sense of history requires us to document a life.
5. A sense of history inspires respect and awareness that other persons' stories are as valid as our own.

Thus, whatever oral and narrative tradition is selected as the basis for conducting an oral history, qualitative researchers may be comfortable with the tried-and-true techniques of the field. Also, oral historians, like all qualitative researchers, need to describe and explain their purposes, their theoretical frames for the study, their methods, and their approaches to analysis and interpretation. We acknowledge that there is no one way to do oral history or qualitative work but that there are many guidelines, practices, and traditions. These are continually discussed and debated and added to our knowledge base.

PERSPECTIVES

I bring various philosophies into the discussion. First, my view of history is that history is both a process and a point of view. What we study is dynamic and, in terms of the postmodernist outlook, is affected by outlook, experience, and reinterpretation of a given experience. I hope to provide a critical perspective to the study of oral history. As discussed in the preface, I have been influenced by the writings of critical pedagogists Freire, Giroux, Kincheloe, Steinberg, and Macedo, to want to bring oral history to life. As someone who started out studying John Dewey's (1859–1952) writings on experience as education, art as experience, and democracy and education, I see my work as an extension of those ideas. I like to think of my work and that of all of us as placed along the continuum of the history of ideas and that we all take part in extending those ideas as we publish our research and interpretation of research. I would have to say that oral history is a type of revisiting of experience, and so a type of educative activity. I see history as a method in and of itself and interpretation as both a goal and a benefit of studying oral history methods. Oral history is also dialogical. I think it is important to illuminate the importance of that fact. Both the researcher and the researched are active in oral history. Oral history is about the excitement and engagement of some lived experience. Oral history validates subjectivity and embraces it. Oral history can be a key element in documenting stories of those on the periphery of society. Thus it validates a multicultural and diverse approach to documenting the lived experience of individuals and groups and becomes an important path to social justice. Qualitative work in general in this, the postmodern, era often raises questions of a social justice nature.

ORAL HISTORY AS A SOCIAL JUSTICE PROJECT

If we take a view of oral history as a social justice project, think of all the potential and possibility. Individuals who may have been overlooked in traditional projects may now have the opportunity to have a voice. Not only that, but we may also all learn from those on the outside of the mainstream. We may learn more about the human condition all the way around. By learning about the lives, ways of knowing, culture, speech, and behavior of those on the periphery of society, we stand to learn more about our society as a whole and more about ourselves as individuals. In fact, we may become more reflexive as we come to understand the perspectives of another. In terms of actually doing oral history, majority members of society may help equalize the record by conducting oral histories of those members traditionally left out of the written record.

Another side of social justice and oral history is the potential for recording the stories of protected populations, such as disabled persons, prisoners, individuals with mental problems, and quite possibly selected children. Overall, each person has a story to tell. It is the work of the oral historian to craft the narratives from the recorded memories of those in a given oral history project. Most recently, testimony given by truth commissions continues to be a good example of oral history for social justice. If we view the case of South Africa and its truth commissions, we see that we have much to learn about this matter. This is not to overlook other truth commissions, such as those in Central or South America, but the South African example offers a unique approach and perspective to testimony as oral history because of its public nature and its focus on reconciliation.

ON THE CRITICAL IMPORTANCE OF TESTIMONY AS ORAL HISTORY

One of the useful prototypes of oral history is testimony. Globally, testimony has been used to document the stories of victims and those perpetrators who committed crimes against them in various parts of Africa and Central America, for example. Testimony of individuals allowed a written record of a catalogue of misdeeds, which then facilitated some measure of social justice. Most often, those victimized faced their perpetrators in court. To use a prime example, let us consider the case of South Africa and the Truth and Reconciliation Commission (TRC). The TRC was a vehicle for capturing the witnesses' stories of the events occurring in South Africa under the then system of apartheid. Obviously, there have been many truth commissions throughout history, beginning with Nuremberg. I focus on the case of South Africa because it is still so close in time to our own experience. It is fresh in the annals of history, and numerous books, such as Desmond Tutu's (1999), are a result of the TRC. Testimony in the case of South Africa allows all of us to more fully understand the political, cultural, emotional, psychological, and social justice aspects of apartheid as never before. Because Africa retains storytelling as part of its culture, the brave individuals who took part in the TRC testimony gave straightforward descriptions, often emotional, of what had occurred while facing those who had committed crimes against them. The perpetrators and victims publicly acknowledged events, which then became the first step toward reconciliation. In fact, Desmond Tutu (1999) has argued that one cannot arrive at forgiveness without factual truth and data as a starting point. Tutu and other writers often catalogue **four types of truth**:

1. **Factual and forensic truth**, that is, the actual evidence of what occurred, such as number of beatings, murders, and violent crimes and where they took place.

2. **Personal or narrative truth**, that is, the person's story and narrative of how something occurred, as well as what occurred and the effect that had on the individual and the family.

3. **Social or cultural truth**, that is, basically, the social context and history of what occurred; in this case, the genesis, activities, development, and sustenance of problems of apartheid.

4. **Healing or restorative truth**, that is, what is needed to heal the wounds uncovered by the engagement with the three previously listed types of truth. When victims faced the perpetrators in court in testimony, the perpetrators had to admit what they had done in order to apply for amnesty. In this instance, South Africa did something no one had seen before, for no blanket amnesty was granted. In addition, the TRC was a public forum, unlike previous commissions.

The power of testimony is simply that people are allowed to tell their stories. Usually, the people in question have had their voices either erased or diminished prior to the testimony. In fact, some testimony providers had no voice whatsoever in the political or social arena. Thus testimony as oral history opens up society to new ways of knowing history. This history may have been completely unavailable to the public had there been no testimony at all. In the case of South Africa, during the testimony of the TRC, all testimony was public, a unique characteristic. In previous truth commissions, in Africa or elsewhere, this was not the case. Everything took place behind closed doors.

Likewise, the South African TRC granted amnesty to select perpetrators under specified conditions and regularly granted compensation to victims in specific cases. What the South African TRC offers us is a living example of how oral history may be used as a social justice project through testimony. Testimony such as that of the survivors of apartheid may emerge as a key element in oral history as a social justice project.

In addition, everyday testimonials are also critical to our understanding and practice of social justice. See this example of Leona, an African American female who participated in my oral history project on women leaders. I am using lengthy sections of the narrative because it helps to capture the voice of the person in question. It is impossible to do a short oral history or even a brief excerpt, and so I hope the reader will agree to read each excerpted example in its entirety.

CASE I.1.
∽

An Excerpt from an Oral History Narrative

Toward Becoming an Educator: A Journey of Self-Discovery—
The Story of Leona M. Graham, in Response to the Statement
"Describe Yourself and Your Work."

Every journey has a beginning, and—although I didn't realize it back then—my journey toward becoming an educator began the day I awoke to realize that I was trapped in a deathbed of my own making, hopeless, alone, and just waiting to die. At 450 pounds I had become extremely depressed, lonely, and isolated. I spent most of my days lazing in bed, watching TV and eating junk food. At the time, I was living in seclusion in a small trailer on an isolated stretch of land on a Pacific Northwest mountain range. My doctors told me that the various health problems I had (e.g., asthma, diabetes, hypertension) were directly related to my morbid obesity. And although I faithfully consumed the medicines they administered to me, I had very little faith in their ability to sustain my life.

On reflection I don't rightfully know if it was an epiphany, or just opportunity knocking, and I don't suppose that it really matters which, because whatever it was I am surely glad that I pursued it when I did. One morning as I lay in bed, my torso propped up on several pillows to help me breathe, I was thumbing through a free newspaper I had picked up at one of the doctors' offices I had recently visited. Tears were burning my eyes as I lifted my head to take a look around my bedroom. Cluttering my nightstand were 12 pill bottles, a nebulizer, a couple of inhalers and a CPAP [continuous positive airway pressure] machine to help me breathe during the night. I had become, in a relatively short period of time, indoctrinated in some morbid sickly daily routine. Each morning I took a pill for my diabetes and a couple of pills for my high blood pressure, a pill for my asthma, and then there was another pill that I took for my high cholesterol, too. Throughout the day I also took iron supplements and daily vitamins and minerals as well. My asthma management regimen also consisted of both metered-dose inhalers and periodic treatments using the nebulizer. I didn't particularly have faith in these medicines—I didn't believe they would make a difference in my life. But I was willing to give them a try nonetheless. Blurry-eyed and feeling hopeless, I slowly thumbed through the newspaper, half-heartedly searching for a new distraction. I wanted something to keep my mind off of my illnesses. I had long grown tired of watching movies, and I was having difficulty concentrating on anything other than my thoughts of being so sick and so fat. When there, on one of the pages of the newspaper, was a 4-inch advertisement about a distance-learning program at a state university.

I hadn't necessarily been thinking about returning to school, because I had no particular desire to ever reenter the workforce. Besides, I didn't think I would be alive long enough to realistically carve out a substantial new career for myself. But I told myself that I needed some sort of distraction during my long days in bed. Sadly, I had dropped out of college years ago, vowing to return to school again someday. But obtaining a college degree had remained one of many promises to me that I had not kept. Nevertheless, I figured that it wouldn't hurt to get more information about this distance-learning program. I liked the idea of being able to get an education from the sanctuary of my home. This way, I reasoned, I could continue to avoid contact with others, being that I was so embarrassed by my weight and all. So I phoned the toll-free number in the newspaper advertisement and within a few weeks my financial aid was in place and I was enrolled in the bachelor's degree program as a full-time student.

One of the three courses I took during that first semester was in women's studies, titled "Gender in Cross-Cultural Perspective." There were a dozen or so videotapes that arrived at my home at the beginning of the semester, along with the syllabus and course assignments for each class. Each of the videotapes contained a 2-hour prerecorded class lecture to accompany the reading assignment for each class session during that semester. The first required reading assignment in that course forever changed my life. Marjorie Shostak's anthropological classic, *Nisa: The Life and Words of a !Kung Woman*, connected with me in a way that is somewhat hard for me to describe, even today. Truthfully, I don't know what it is about Nisa and her intimate story of being a !Kung woman in her early 50s, living in the Kalahari Desert, that seemed to resonate so powerfully with me. Perhaps it was the tribe's isolation; perhaps it was the harsh environment; perhaps it was Nisa's victimization or her strong will to survive. Maybe it was a combination of several factors concerning that story, who knows? But whatever it was, as I journeyed with Nisa, I felt stronger about the possibility of overcoming my own illnesses, both physical and emotional.

I also believe the instructor for the course was undeniably instrumental in making a real difference in my life. She, too, seemed to embody a sort of resiliency and determination to succeed that instantly captured my attention and admiration. And I immediately noticed a difference in the way that I viewed myself and in the way I perceived my value as a human being. Whatever it was, it worked! On the first day of class, at the beginning of the introductory video, the professor told the viewing audience a little bit about herself. She, too, had returned to school as an older student to pursue a degree. Initially she hadn't planned on becoming an educator. She had experienced some difficulties as a younger learner, too. The way I remember it, she also seemed to poke fun at her own weight problem and appearance, and yet she seemed to be delightfully at ease with her rounded body, thinning hair, and older age. Her clothing was somewhat outdated but looked extremely comfortable and appropriate for her body size. She didn't wear makeup, but she was fond of adorning her ears and neckline with jewelry that looked Native American or Mexican in origin. Her speaking style was soothing and reassuring to me. Her real appeal, I think, was that she taught class with an amazingly relaxed method of communicating. She presented material and permitted us to make sense of it in any way we wished. And as I watched her on tape I remember thinking, "Wow, what a self-affirming career choice; I bet I could one day do this, too." And at that instant, I pictured myself one day teaching a class and using my life experiences to help others along their way.

I ended up watching that videotape for that first class several more times, just because it felt so good to hear the professor recount her triumph over her past struggles in school and problems in life. Seemingly she acknowledged some of the common challenges that one faces in juggling schoolwork with the responsibilities of family life and a job. She encouraged us to stick with the distance-learning program and to not give up when things inevitably got tough. Surprisingly, she also required us to begin journaling as a means of communication and gaining personal insight, which I admittedly hadn't done in years! Each day I diligently wrote a little bit more in my journal. And in doing so, I immediately seemed to begin connecting the dots, so to speak, in the areas of my life that previously seemed befuddled, severed, and amorphous. Then I would rewatch the videotapes again. And as the professor spoke, week after week, I became more comfortable in my own skin and with my own struggles.

Once I started to accept the possibility of my own recovery, I began searching for assistance to help me in other areas of my life. For instance, I bought some workout videos to help me establish a daily exercise routine. I joined a study group to enhance my understanding of course materials. I searched for online information and Internet support groups for the various diagnoses I had been given. And I sought counseling to help me deal with the layers of emotional turmoil and cognitive dissonance that had originally caused me to isolate myself and turn to food for comfort. In no time at all, I was feeling alive again, and I wanted to do everything in my power to live well and to live long. So I moved back to the city and began interacting with people again. In time I shed about 250 pounds. As a result, I no longer had to sleep with a CPAP machine. I no longer had diabetes or high blood pressure or asthma or high cholesterol, either. They all disappeared with the extra weight. Going back to school and learning more about myself made me a healthier person—both inside and out.

My journey to becoming an educator is inextricably linked to my journey of self-discovery and physical–emotional recovery. In time I was able to begin integrating myself with others. As I lost weight, I gained confidence. Eventually I was even comfortable with sitting in a classroom with other students. After I received my bachelor of arts degree, I went on to earn a master of science in marriage and family therapy. I chose this field because I wanted to help other people who may have experienced similar life crises. Once I became a therapist, I was able to help hundreds of individuals from various walks of life as they struggled with emotional problems and serious mental illness. I treated dozens of women like myself, who had turned to food or alcohol or drugs or sex or whatever in dealing with their depression. Many of them had become isolated or had cocooned themselves in one type of addiction or another in an effort to cope with their feelings of loss, guilt, helplessness, and/or hopelessness. I provided them with individual and group therapy in order to help them discover for themselves the keys to their own recovery and self-awareness. In addition, I conducted workshops to help both women and men manage the symptoms of their various emotional problems.

I eventually accepted a position as bicultural specialist at the community mental health center where I had been working as a therapist. It was in this capacity that I discovered an affinity for teaching. As a bicultural specialist, it was my responsibility to provide training and consultation to fellow mental health care clinicians in the area of multicultural services and cross-cultural treatment. On several occasions I was asked to speak to large groups of practitioners in an effort to teach them how to provide culturally relevant and appropriate treatment interventions to mental health care consumers from various ethnic groups. In doing so, I discovered that I had a natural talent for engaging the audience and connecting with my "students" in a meaningful way.

My success as a trainer led me to decide to continue my education in order to acquire the necessary tools I would need in becoming an agent of change in the mental health care industry overall. My goal was to help change the way that mental health care professionals are trained in the area of working with minority mental health care consumers and ethnically different clientele. So I packed up my belongings and moved 2,000 miles away to become a doctoral student in an educational leadership program at a university in Chicago, Illinois. Soon after arriving in Chicago, I accepted a job position in the psychiatric rehabilitation field at a major university, as part of a training team charged with the responsibility of developing curricula and conducting training for paraprofessionals who are providing treatment for individuals with serious mental illness.

A large part of my job on the psychiatric rehabilitation training team is focused on training mental health care providers on how to engage their clients (or patients) to participate in the treatment process. Most recently I have dedicated my time to training staff members employed at long-term-care facilities (i.e., nursing homes). The focus of my attention is specifically devoted to training staff at the facilities that provide residency for individuals who suffer from pervasive and serious mental illnesses. These illnesses range in scope from depression to schizophrenia and, understandably, can become extremely disabling to the residents at these facilities. Generally speaking, the paraprofessional staff members at these facilities have relatively very little formal training. Many of them possess only a high school education. Some have merely an eighth-grade equivalency. Staff burnout is quite common. Staff turnover is so high in these facilities that employees generally don't hang around long enough to participate in rigorous continuing education programs. And once on duty, they generally don't have the luxury of having extra staff on hand to cover the floor so that they may take an afternoon away from their duties in order to attend an extensive training session. So my team members and I have discovered that short-term training series involving a combination of 1-hour interactive sessions and on-site learning exercises (e.g., role playing at the nurses' station) tend to be most successful in this busy, demanding environment.

The employees at these kinds of facilities often feel frustrated about their inability to motivate the residents of these facilities to care for themselves. According to the staff, many of the residents seem unmotivated to get out of bed, to take their medicine, or to set goals toward their own recovery and eventual discharge from the facility. Fortunately, I recognize a lot of the apathy that these residents appear to be feeling. I know firsthand how easy it is to become depressed, hopeless, and even self-destructive. Like the residents in these long-term-care facilities, at one time I too felt unmotivated to get out of bed. I remember the days when I didn't have much faith in the efficacy of medical treatment. And I also know what it takes to overcome painful past experiences in life in order to prevail. So I use my intimate knowledge of depression, along with my education and experience as a therapist, in an effort to provide insight to the staff members at the long-term-care facilities on how they might be successful in helping the residents recover.

It is tremendously rewarding for me to be able to help these staff members be successful in their jobs. More so, it is rewarding for me to be instrumental in providing treatment (albeit vicariously) to individuals with serious mental illness. These individuals are often forgotten and easily overlooked in our nation's health care system riddled with budgetary constraints, managed care, and a scarcity of available professionals willing to take on these tough cases. It isn't easy working with individuals who suffer from pervasive mental health problems. But research indicates that through the application of current best practices in providing clinical care and case management for these people, many of the problems associated with their mental illnesses can be successfully reduced, managed, and often even prevented. One important way to effect change within these long-term-care facilities is to develop skills among staff members and among the residents themselves. And this is what our training and curricula are designed to do: (a) teach staff new skills, and (b) teach staff how to teach residents new skills toward recovery and symptom management.

I try to keep the curricular materials as user friendly as possible, keeping in mind that the reader may feel overworked, underpaid, and unappreciated (a.k.a. burned out). Working in a long-term-care environment is extremely difficult to do. It becomes even more difficult when one is expected to add to the existing workload by trying to teach residents new psychosocial skills that the residents themselves may not necessarily wish to learn. Consequently, the training materials that I produce are purposely designed to provide a basic understanding of psychosocial rehabilitation through the use of simple language and easy-to-understand PowerPoint presentations. I also try to remember that when presenting the content of the material, it is important to use the level of language being used by the staff members who are being trained at the facilities. It is hoped that this will, in turn, model for staff members how they, too, should use the level of language used by the residents who they will in turn be training. Otherwise, both the staff members and the residents are likely to reject psychosocial rehabilitation (along with my training materials) as being too lofty a concept or too difficult to grasp.

Of chief importance, I do my best to make the training experience contextually based. To be effective, I believe the learning process has to mean something to the training participants. Otherwise it isn't authentic, and it isn't going to stick. As such, I carefully incorporate real-life examples and exercises that make sense in both the paraprofessionals' world and in the world of the individuals who reside in the long-term-care facilities. This I have found to be most significant in engaging the learner during training sessions. You have got to keep it real!

At the time of this interview and writing, I am entering my final semester in the program. Once completed, I will write my dissertation, graduate, and then continue my journey as a lifelong learner. At this point I plan to spend the next decade continuing my research and writing in the area of best practices in psychiatric rehabilitation, teaching mental health care practitioners who are working with individuals with mental illness. I believe I have a unique perspective as an educational leader in the mental health care field because I've been on the "other side of the fence," so to speak. I've also had the honor of accompanying many individuals as they journeyed to their own psychiatric recoveries.

On a personal level, I will soon celebrate my first-year wedding anniversary with my husband, whom I met shortly after arriving in Chicago. He has consistently been my biggest cheerleader and source of emotional support and encouragement. He's a remarkable man with a fascinating and inspirational recovery story of his own. Our newborn is a joy to come home to. She helps me to laugh, to relax, and to just be in the moment (which is something that I admit with which I still have some struggle). Nevertheless, I am having fun being an educator at the parenting level now, too. With Lisa, I continue to experience a lot of self-discovery for myself as I interact with her and as I observe her grow and develop. Above all else, my prayer for her is that she will be a strong and independent female. I never want her to be afraid to take a chance, to leap, or to dance. I feel blessed to have been the one chosen to guide her and to help her spirit soar. I am very excited about taking this journey alongside Lisa.

Indeed, there is something magical about being an educator. I don't think the magic can be found in how we teach or what we teach . . . or even necessarily who we teach. To me, the magic exists in our willingness to walk that gentle journey alongside an active learner, no matter how long that journey may take. As an educator I feel spiritually whole, emotionally fulfilled, and physically strong when I take that learning journey with another individual. When I have the privilege of accompanying the learner on his or her personal journey, the destination is of little or no consequence because it is the experience of the journey that I find most rewarding. I tend to think of being an educator as being a willing participant in a reciprocal process in which I may teach, but I consequently also learn so much more! Perhaps that is the real magic of being an educator—committing oneself to being a co-learner rather than having to be the trailblazer or tour guide all the time. For me, as I think about the journey I took in getting to where I am today, I am reminded of all that I had to learn about myself in order to be able to help others. Mind you, my journey is far from being over. I still have much to learn. And I look forward to doing so. Truthfully, I really enjoy being a co-learner in life. In essence, what I truly treasure about my journey thus far is not necessarily the stuff I gleaned from books but how I utilized the experiences in my life, along with the experiences in the lives of others, in order to know which path in life to take next.

The reader can see the power of oral history techniques in this example. You may be happy to know that, since the completion of that oral history project, Leona has achieved her goal of completing and earning a doctorate and has started her own company consulting in her field. Her history can be seen as part of the mosaic of oral history as a social justice project. In terms of social justice, she is a minority female once also marginalized because of her weight. Now she has come into balance and redirected her story. This brings up another important value of oral history: the fact that an oral history of an individual may provide hope, inspiration, and transformation for those reading the narrative. Readers of an oral history may find something in the narrative to inspire them and even stand as a model for them, as an additional bonus. In fact, I hope that oral history as a qualitative research technique will be considered in my own field, education, and in others related to the field of history as a worthwhile research approach. Now is a good time to document stories of educators who have stories to tell. Currently, in education, we are experiencing one of the great debates that often take place when the public sphere is under critique. As high-stakes testing and one-size-fits-all technocratic measures of testing are hotly debated, we need to get at the reasons for the sharp divisions in the field of education. Educators and educational researchers do use other narrative approaches from time to time. Hopefully, oral history methods will help a great deal in documenting this time of debate, dissent, and occasional acrimony.

Of course, this example of a narrative is written in the voice of the narrator and provides us with a good example of understanding the narrator's story. Another technique that oral historians and other qualitative researchers use to their advantage is observation. We can use observation to set a context, to describe that context, and to place the narrator in a specific context. I use an observation activity in my research class, which is described in Appendix L. I have students train themselves to be better observers by going to a public setting at least twice and describing it. Then they need to try to connect what they observe to some of the history and social context of whatever it is they are observing. The following case example is well written, and I use it to point out the power of observation. Like the choreographer who has to tell a story within a context, a researcher in training has to, as well.

CASE I.2.
༒

Observing in Spring Hill Cemetery
BY JODY J. JAMISON

This study is based on observations completed at the Spring Hill Cemetery, aka Brooksville Civil War Cemetery, located just off Fort Dade Avenue, between Brooksville and Spring Hill in Hernando County, Florida. Prior to this assignment, I had not visited this cemetery, although I had heard rumors of paranormal activity at the gravesites. Though not a fan of paranormal activity, I am interested in cemeteries as locations of historical artifacts. Sadly, Hernando County is rife with documented accounts of human atrocities and unspeakable acts of violence. While also known for its strategic role in the Civil War, Hernando County's rich history is overshadowed by reports of abuse and tragedy of a marginalized community of African Americans.

In this report, I will take you on a tour of Hernando County's history as we pass through the Spring Hill Cemetery and unearth stories that lie buried deeply beneath the layers of a community that screams out for justice. Even though no one visited the cemetery during the times I conducted my observations, I believe I was able to observe the citizens of a lost community through the small, unassuming artifacts left behind in the form of grave markers. By observing these remnants of a community, I gained a new appreciation for close examination. Though I could not observe movements of people as they maneuvered through a room, I did observe movements of people as their gravesites were carefully positioned into patterns; though I could not observe expressions as people looked at one another in conversation, I could observe the print on the grave markers telling me whether a child or adult lay beneath; though I could not observe hand or facial gestures, I could observe the angst of frustration of broken lives reflected in small, unmarked stones left unclaimed and untended. Therefore, I believe my observations rendered data about a community whose voices can no longer be hushed.

Located just off Fort Dade Avenue in Brooksville, Florida, the cemetery lies isolated from the main community. Although the cemetery is also known as the Brooksville Civil War Cemetery, very few Civil War soldiers are buried there. Rather, it houses a Black community, many of whom were victims of brutal lynchings between 1900 and 1930. A website called *Ghostvillage.com* hosts ghost research, evidence, and discussion and is home to lively conversations from people who claim to have seen spectral residents of Spring Hill Cemetery.

THE COMMUNITY OF SPRING HILL CEMETERY: THE SETTING

Fort Dade Avenue, the road off which Spring Hill Cemetery is located, begins like most any other small, two-lane, rural road. It is a long road that extends from the east end of the county to the west, bridging the two communities of Brooksville and Spring Hill. Shortly after crossing Cobb Road, a two-lane road dividing Fort Dade Avenue into east and west sections, the scenery quickly changes. Massive and regal oak trees bend into the shape of an arch by a natural phenomenon known as the Florida Hammocks. As I drive west on Fort Dade Avenue, I feel as if I were entering a different world. Traffic is nearly nonexistent, the sky disappears behind a dense mass of green, and sounds draw near as the

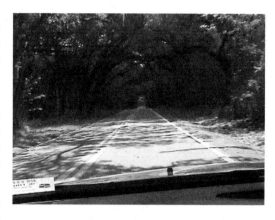

trees trap them near to the ground. Nature is so close; I can feel it as I put my hand outside the window, and smell it as it fills my car.

Consistent with the humble lives of those residing in the cemetery, a simple green sign announces the entrance. After a few feet of roadway, the lane transforms into dirt and sugar sand, making it difficult to avoid getting trapped. Invisible from Fort Dade Avenue, nothing draws attention to the community residing at the end of the winding dirt road. Large oak trees border the lane, and the sounds of crickets and birds accompany me on the journey. Nature abounds along the entrance; no attention has been given to the area by road crews or county maintenance. The grass remains untended, allowing weeds and underbrush to flourish. Signs of disrespect—a filthy mattress, a broken chair—line the diminutive lane leading to the cemetery. Trash is strewn as bottles, paper plates, and plastics gather into piles under the oak trees. The oaks, many of which are several feet in diameter, are largely free of the Spanish moss for which they are so famous. The smell of walnut trees— sharp, and yet mellow, but distinctly different from oaks—pierces the air. The air is dry and hot. Each of the two cars that drive by as I examine the entrance leaves a cyclone of dust that floats in the air for several minutes after they pass. I think it ironic how the floating dust parallels the lives of those I would soon visit—living in a flurry, floating in the air for several moments as they pass.

Returning to my car, I venture into the cemetery. The oak trees, once tightly connected and overlapping one another at the entrance, now open as a welcoming gesture to an unfamiliar visitor. Spanish moss, nonexistent on the entrance oaks, now wraps the lane in a boa of grey flannel. Lowering my car windows, I notice how quiet this site is;

the trees make a slight sound as their tiny leaves chatter in the wind. The sound of a passing vehicle makes a distant whirring noise. The smells of oak and walnut provoke thoughts about an old Florida—an antebellum Florida— which incites memories of a book I read, entitled *A Land Remembered*, that depicts the life of cattle rustling in an antebellum Florida where beach property is useless because of its inability to produce crops. Life depended on practicality; thus I am once again reminded of how that relates to the residents of

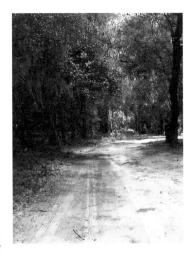

Spring Hill Cemetery. Their lives, too, often depended on practicality.

Once again forcing myself to focus on the purpose of this visit, I prepare to observe my host setting. As the density of great oak trees begins to thin, I see the first signs of the cemetery community. The first grave marker stands taller than any other in the cemetery. Appearing as if to have at one time housed a plaque or nameplate, the brick enclosure is now empty. Three smaller markers lying beneath the tall monument contain the nearly invisible names of their residents. These small white stones lie just behind it, yet remain anonymous. The only marker whose writing remains legible contains the name Pearl Mobley; however, the date embossed below is too faded to read.

As I walk in this community, I feel an obligation to carefully avoid stepping on the lives buried beneath. My plastic Crocs tentatively step across the terrain, crunching dry grass and dead leaves as they echo

in the absence of all other sound. I no longer hear the chattering leaves of the oak trees that greeted me as I entered the cemetery; I no longer hear the crickets and birds that accompanied my journey down the dusty lane that brought me to this community. Only the sounds of my footsteps exist.

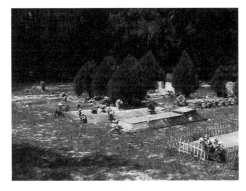

Unlike some cemeteries where the only marker is that of the monument, many of the Spring Hill Cemetery plots contain above-ground burials. Something I find particularly interesting is that the above-ground sites are enclosed in what appear to be concrete structures rather than marble ones, and some of them have been sprayed with grey metallic paint to resemble a metal container. While the paint makes it difficult to read the inscriptions, it appears to resist black mold that covers some of the unpainted tombs.

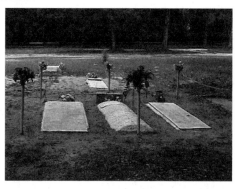

The family plots, in particular, are maintained with plastic and silk flowers. Some are enclosed with white picket fences; others are enclosed by chains. Very little grass grows in the cemetery, and some family plots are dotted with sprigs of grass, while others appear to be completely free of any grass. Only the fallen leaves of the giant oak trees carpet the ground surrounding the graves and provide a path for visitors to follow.

Close to the cemetery entrance stands a tall oak tree bent over at the top. Beneath is a white cross marking it as, according to some, the "hanging tree," where Black men were lynched. Because of the isolated location of the cemetery, atrocities could go unnoticed by the towns-

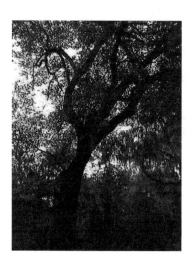

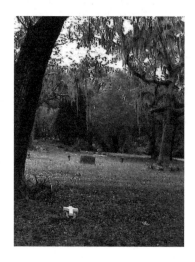

people. Archival records likewise corroborate that this location served as a meeting place for the Ku Klux Klan in the 1920s and 1930s. The tree thus stands as a monument, much like the grave markers, that speaks to the lives of Spring Hill Cemetery's residents and to the shame of a county that conceded to the will of unsavory leaders.

OBSERVATION 1

A tiny grave marker rests on its side as if it were intentionally placed in this position so visitors could read its message. Shaped like a park bench, with two tiny footstools as its support, it now rests on its side. A beautiful angel wearing a pale green and pink gown floating over raised, white clouds graces the marker. A black metal plate is embedded into a ridge of flowers encircling it; however, what was written has since been lost to the natural elements. My inclination is to set the marker upright; but I pull my hand back, as it is not my place to correct anything in this community. Perhaps the marker's position was intentionally changed; perhaps it would be a sign of disrespect for a visitor to impose her sense of balance and proportion on a community that survived the greatest example of imbalance and disproportion imposed upon it by those who thought they should make changes. So I leave this little marker while I imagine the tiny resident it represents.

As I walk a few paces, I am drawn to a most shy resident, as I notice the marker heavily burdened by mold that serves to obscure its name. Identified only as "Edmund," this resident informs me of its birth in 1831 and its death in 1901; it boasts a long life of 70 years, some of which no doubt witnessed the brutalities imposed upon its friends and family by ruthless people inflamed by ugly and unjust hatred. Many markers share characteristics with that of Edmund. Carved from marble, shaped into rectangular posts, they show the wear of time and proclaim their presence in quiet dignity.

An even shier resident marks its place in the cemetery, yet keeps its name a mystery. A simple stone that marks the place where a life once existed sits quietly just beyond where Edmund's rests. Betraying no concern for fanfare or remembrance, the grave marker serves only to announce that a resident lies here.

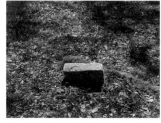

One of the most intriguing grave markers is that of "Mammie," B—5/5/1895, D—5/30/1953. Carved by hand, the marker appears to be homemade. Seemingly molded from concrete, it rests at the head of approximately 15 ceramic tiles of varying colors, creating a most unique gravesite. It is unclear whether Mammie's last name is Delaine, or if Delaine is the person who crafted the marker. Nonetheless, it makes me curious how Mammie, a 58-year-old woman, came to reside here.

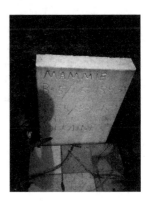

OBSERVATION 2

Upon my return for the second observation, the road is a bit more difficult to drive on because of a storm the previous evening. As I near the cemetery, I notice a silver pickup truck with the logo of the State Forestry Department on its doors exiting the cemetery very slowly, most likely checking for signs of illegal activity. Since beginning this project, I have learned that the Spring Hill Cemetery is frequented by drug dealers; so both state and local officials regularly sweep the area. I find it perplexing, however, that of the many state and local officials who apparently sweep the area for illegal activities, not one local or state official deems it worthy to remove the trash and other man-made debris from the cemetery's community.

Today, I focus on individuals in the cemetery community. One grave marker catches my eye because it contains a photograph of a woman identified as Retha Timmons. That name interests me because of its history. According to a July 5, 2005, article in the *St. Petersburg Times*, journalist Dan DeWitt reports that in 1924, Retha Timmons's uncle, Will Timmons, a "prosperous black farmer . . . bought a new car. . . . As she returned with him from the fields, he was confronted by a group of white men . . . and then beaten 'half to death'." The article likewise reported statements from people who were familiar with the incident, and one person reported that "the mob beat (Timmons) between the legs until they tore his testicles up. . . . They did castrate him because he bought a brand-new Ford." Will's grave lies just to the left of Waiters

Timmons and to the right of Retha Timmons, as if he is now under the protection of beloved sentries.

REFLECTIONS ABOUT THE SETTING
AND MY APPROACH TO THIS PROJECT

If I had all the time in the world to observe this site, I would list the names of all residents from their grave markers and try to find out who they were. Even though there may no longer be sanctioned lynchings in Brooksville, there still remain dramatic inequalities. Most of Brooksville's Black population lives off of Summit Avenue (now called Martin Luther King Blvd.). Their community has recently been the subject of an Environmental Protection Agency investigation because the old Hernando County Public Works Department dumped toxic waste in the creek behind the complex, which in turn feeds into the Black community's drinking water. After the incident became public, medical teams investigated what appeared to be unusually high infant mortality rates and deaths among children in the Black community along Martin Luther King Blvd. Yet, after a flurry of investigations, no changes have been made—no improvements, no restitutions, no fulfilled promises— as a legal or symbolic gesture by the county. In the recent past, county commissioners have felt an obligation to make a formal apology to the Black community for past atrocities; however, that apology has rarely, if ever, been accompanied by funding or community improvements.

What I would like to be able to do with the information I accumulate is, at the very least, use it to motivate the county commission to provide groundskeeping services for the Spring Hill Cemetery—if the Black community so wishes. But, if the county provides so little assistance to living residents, I am doubtful they will find it within their budgets or interests to provide assistance to the dead. Nonetheless, it is the choice of the Black community whether they want their loved ones to be bothered by county workers whose ancestors were, in part, responsible for populating the Spring Hill Cemetery community. This project attempted also to use photos to tell a story. In accord with Freirian philosophy, we all have the responsibility to advocate for the many who have neither the voice nor the opportunity to advocate for themselves, even if this means that we look to the dead for stories that often speak louder than words of the living.

As I examined community lives in the Spring Hill Cemetery, I realized that this activity shares characteristics of an oral history project. Likewise, my observations of past lives in the Spring Hill Cemetery through trying to understand gravestones and markers could contribute to a social justice project that repairs Hernando County's historical record by including voices from the Black community.

Perhaps the very best argument of all for my approach in this project is that it functions as a creative tool through which others may access past events. Creativity is imperative to counteract—if only symbolically—the effects of past actions inflicted upon a community.

SELF-REFLECTION

Needless to say, this assignment has left me with more questions than answers, and the precious few answers I do have have led me to more questions. Thus there is a circularity to qualitative research—a cycle that is perpetually fueled by inquiry. Though I was unable to observe a visitor to the Spring Hill Cemetery during this assignment, I believe this itself is an observation that leads me to ask: Where are the families? Where are the visitors? While working on this assignment, I drifted into the Brooksville Cemetery, which houses predominantly White residents. The grass is green, lush, and well maintained; a paved lane meanders through the cemetery, providing ample space for visitors to park and walk. Even the oldest grave marker, which dates to the early 1800s, is clean and free of mold. Trees are trimmed and clear of Spanish moss. On both days I glanced into the White cemetery, there were a number of people visiting grave sites, and I once again wonder: Why are there no visitors in the Spring Hill Cemetery?

As I consider this question, I realize that the Spring Hill Cemetery is located in a remote section of Hernando County, several miles from the Black community. Relatively few people—especially people who are old enough to remember the residents of the cemetery—have transportation. For those who do have transportation, the visit to Spring Hill Cemetery may be dangerous. The road leading to the cemetery, Fort Dade Avenue, is often patrolled by law enforcement trolling for illegal drug activity. Law enforcement has not been kind to Hernando County's Black community in the past, and there remains a tension between law enforcement and the Black community even today. The taken-for-granted privilege of visiting the dead in our cemeteries is most often a White privilege, not a Black one.

Observing people in a social environment can render untold amounts of data; it can help us see the nuances of a person's personality through gestures, facial expressions, and body language. Observations prompt us to ask questions about what we see and what we do not see. Interestingly, it is often what we do not see that renders the most compelling data. As a species, humans have become very clever at creating the image they want others to see. However, they cannot mask that which cannot be readily seen, and this, for me, is the most fertile area to begin observations. Spring Hill Cemetery provided me with abundant data that has left pages of unanswered questions. Some of those questions can be answered by examining archival data; but others can be answered only by talking with people familiar with the person or incident in question.

Racial inequality and tensions continue to plague the United States, and my observations for this assignment have led me to believe that Hernando County, Florida, is an excellent site for researching the ways in which the past continues to guide what happens in the present. Though there exist many well-intentioned White people in Hernando County who are ashamed of its role in racial atrocities, they often mistakenly believe a political apology, a plaque in honor of a Black resident, or a street named in honor of a civil rights leader will set matters right. These White residents do not see that they continue to show disrespect to the Black community when they, for example, vote to discontinue bus service in the county to save money (as they have recently done) without calculating how this will affect a community with no personal transportation. They do not see how their actions complicate the lives of Black citizens when they wholeheartedly support road improvements that require Black children to cross a much wider road to catch a school bus, thus endangering their lives. They do not see how the privileges and conveniences they take for granted every day are inaccessible to the Black community. And they do not understand why the Black community does not appreciate their token apologies for past injustices.

Perhaps the most personally important part of this observation assignment is that it has enlightened me about a community of which I have been a part for nearly 30 years. Having lived in Hernando County longer than I have lived in any other state or county, I realize that I am more intimately attached to the history than I might have originally thought. As I walked the observation site, I recognized many of the names. They were connected to former coworkers, my children's schools, and Little League.

Perhaps paranormal enthusiasts are correct when they say the Spring Hill Cemetery is haunted, for **I am now truly haunted by questions raised during my observation of its residents.** So few questions have been answered about the lives of Black residents in Hernando County; so little is contained in the archival records that would provide those answers; only a handful of people remain who can provide firsthand accounts of Hernando County's history of dealing with the Black community. Therefore, this observation assignment has given me new insight into a community of which I have become a part—a community whose stories are screaming to be heard.

In this example, the writer uses photographs and her narrative style to capture the physical setting but also tries to connect the history of the setting with her narration and with her reflection on Spring Hill Cemetery. I ask learners to identify what they would go back to observe if they had all the time in the world. In this particular example, Jody, the author and observer, would go back to find out more about the history of race relations, although she had started looking for documents before she began. In addition, she was inspired to find documents about the markers she did see but was unsuccessful in finding any records. This to me is another reason to document our various histories.

SUMMARY

Oral history is an age-old technique used to capture personal narratives that represent an individual's or sets of individuals' life stories. As I pointed out earlier, a number of terms are used interchangeably with the term *oral history*. All these approaches use the techniques of the qualitative researcher, which include interview, observation, document review, field notes, journaling, and, more recently, photography and/or photoethnography, digital stories, videotaping of a life or portion of someone's life, and narrative interpretive text in written, spoken, or video format. In this book, interpretation is critical to understanding the story being told. In addition, the importance of testimony as a form of oral history and the use of oral history to include the voices previously silenced are steps toward developing a social justice perspective in oral history projects. An example of testimony as oral history contributing to social justice was provided. In addition, an example of an observation was provided to illustrate the strength of capturing a context and physical setting. In addition, both examples are examples of solid narrative storytelling.

As a suggestion for further study, a visit to a nearby local or university library may surprise you as you search for oral histories. There are many oral histories waiting to be read and reviewed. For example, a recent Web-based library search revealed numerous oral histories in the Tampa Bay area alone. Also found was the Samuel Proctor Oral History Program at the University of Florida, Gainesville, a project begun in 1967, which has already collected more than 4,000 oral histories, making it the largest archive in the United States. In this collection, more than 900 interviews with Native Americans, including Seminoles, Creeks, Cherokee, and other nations' members, are available. This collection also contains the stories of African American civil rights activists, of women in Florida, of World War II veterans, and of Florida politicians, among others. I use these examples to suggest that you, the reader, if you should be inspired to continue this kind of work, might do well to check into what is available in your local area and see what types of oral history projects already exist. Because oral history is a qualitative research endeavor, this work may broaden your skill set and provide a vehicle to tell a previously untold story.

Even more astounding are the numbers of oral histories in process and documented on the World Wide Web. A visit to YouTube, Second Life, MySpace, and, in general, any oral history site will yield hundreds of thousands of oral history projects. On YouTube alone, nearly 2.5 million entries were listed recently under "oral histories." Numerous sites connected to the National Archives and other archives are also available on the Web. A list of examples of the many projects available is excerpted in the Appendices. In addition, many websites are totally dedicated to doing and documenting oral histories. All of these are available free and take only your time.

PERFORMANCE EXERCISES

1. Visit your local library and find an oral history or oral history archive. Select one example to read and study. Use this as an example for practicing an oral history interview with someone in your family—a grandparent, aunt, or uncle, for example. Ask them to describe something memorable in each adult decade of their lives. Practice with a digital voice recorder and practice uploading the interview on your thumb drive to a CD for transcription.

2. Complete a transcription of an oral history interview. Read through the transcription carefully and see what themes emerge from the interview. Write three pages about the themes that emerge and what you want to know next about this person.

3. Write three pages describing your own theoretical framework or one big idea that influences your work and/or your life. Try to find the origin of that idea, trace it to yourself, and say something about how you are extending that idea in the history of ideas. For example, if you are a writer who writes with social justice as a theme, can you name who else currently or in the past also used social justice as a guiding theme? (See also Tutu, 1999.)

4. Find an oral history project on the World Wide Web. Select two examples of oral histories and compare and contrast what you see in the interviews. Find three cultural issues raised by these stories. Write three pages reflecting on the implications for social justice emerging from these oral histories.

5. In order to document a setting, go to a public space and observe at least two different times to get a sense of action, setting, and people. Describe it and connect it to a social justice issue. Reflect on this in writing.

WEB RESOURCES

www.oralhistory.org (Oral History Association)
omega.dickinson.edu/organizations/oha
historymatters.gmu.edu/mse/oral
www.dohistory.org/on_your_own/toolkit/oralHistory.html
www.historians.org (American Historical Association)
ohr.oxfordjournals.org (Oral History Review)
www.Studsterkel.org (Studs Terkel, Chicago Historical Society)
www.personalhistorians.org (Association of Personal Historians)
www.loc.gov/vets/about.html (Veterans Oral History Project at the Library of Congress)

Digital Storytelling Sites, Some with How-to-Do History Guides

www.digitales.us
www.storycenter.org
www.historicalvoices.org
www.dohistory.org
www.photovoice.org
www.positiveexposure.org

OTHER RELATED USEFUL RESOURCES
FOR THOSE INTERESTED IN ORAL HISTORY

Armitage, S., Hart, P., & Weathermon, K. (Eds.). (2002). *Women's oral history: The frontiers reader.* Lincoln: University of Nebraska Press.

Boris, E., & Chaudhuri, N. (1999). *Voices of women historians: The personal, the political, the professional.* Bloomington: University of Indiana Press.

Boschma, G., Yonge, O., & Mychajilunow, L. (2003). Consent in oral history interviews: Unique challenges. *Qualitative Health Research, 13*(1), 129–135.

Cosslet, T., Lury, C., & Summerfield, P. (Eds.). (2000). *Feminism and autobiography: Texts, theories, methods.* London: Routledge.

Davis, C., Back, K., & MacLean, K. (1977). *Oral history from tape to type.* Chicago: American Library Association.

Delaplane-Conti, K. (1995). Oral histories: The most overlooked public relations tool. *Communication World, 12*(6), 52–56.

Dunaway, D. K., & Baum, W. K. (1984). *Oral history: An interdisciplinary anthology.* Nashville, TN: American Association for State and Local History and the Oral History Association.

Foley, J. M. (1988). *The theory of oral composition: History and methodology.* Bloomington: University of Indiana Press.

Gardner, P. (2003). Oral history in education: Teacher's memory and teacher history. *History of Education, 32*(2), 175–188.

Gluck, S. B., & Patai, D. (Eds.). (1991). *Women's words: The feminist practice of oral history.* London: Routledge.

Hannay, D. (2002). Oral history and qualitative research. *British Journal of General Practice: The Journal of the Royal College of General Practitioners, 52*(479), 515.

Havlice, P. (1985). *Oral history: A reference guide and annotated bibliography.* Jefferson, NC: McFarland.

Hoopes, J. (1979). *Oral history: An introduction for students.* Chapel Hill: University of North Carolina Press.

Martin, R. (1995). *Oral history in social work: Research, assessment, and intervention.* Thousand Oaks, CA: Sage.

McMahan, E. (1989). *Elite oral history discourse: A study of cooperation and coherence.* Tuscaloosa: University of Alabama Press.

Nevins, A., & Perlstein, S. (1984). Oral histories of women. *Gerontologist, 24*(3), 600–601.

Rafael, A. R. (1997). Advocacy oral history: A research methodology for social activism in nursing. *Methods of Clinical Inquiry, 20*(2), 32–43.

Rubin, H. J., & Rubin, I. S. (2005). *Qualitative interviewing: The art of hearing data.* Thousand Oaks, CA: Sage.

Rumic, E. (1966). Oral history: Defining the term. *Wilson Library Bulletin, 40*(7), 602–603.

Samuel, R., & Thompson, P. (Eds.). (1990). *The myths we live by.* London: Routledge.

Schneider, W. (2002). *So they understand: Cultural issues in oral history.* Logan: Utah State University Press.

Terkel, S. (1984). *The good war: An oral history of World War II.* New York: Ballantine.

Terkel, S. (1986). *Talking to myself: A memoir of my times.* London: Harrap.

Tollefson, J. W. (1993). *The strength not to fight: An oral history of conscientious objections of the Vietnam War.* Boston: Little, Brown.

Walker, M. (Ed.). (2004). *Country women cope with hard times: A collection of oral histories.* Columbia: University of South Carolina Press.

Ward, C. (2000). *Oral histories and analyses of nontraditional women students: A study of unconventional strengths.* New York: Mellen Press.

Wieder, A. (2004). Testimony as oral history: Lessons from South Africa. *Educational Researcher, 33*(6), 23–34.

PART II

~

DESIGN AND TENSION

The Tools of the Oral Historian: The Choreography of Techniques and Issues

Tell me a fact and I'll learn.
Tell me a truth and I'll believe.
But tell me a story and it will live in
My heart forever.
—INDIAN PROVERB

INTRODUCTION

All oral historians, like all qualitative researchers, have to come to grips with the age-old and primary techniques of interviewing and document analysis. In addition, in this, the postmodern era, visual images from photography and videotaping may take prominent roles in terms of technique. Because interviewing is the mainstay of oral history, the discussion begins here. There are literally thousands of articles in print and hundreds of books on interviewing. Obviously, interviewing has taken hold in the social sciences, in the arts and the sciences, in society at large, in business, and in journalism. For

43

the purposes of this book, we look at interviewing in multiple ways. The first way is metaphorically, by conceptualizing an interview much like a choreographer conceptualizes a dance. Both choreographer and interviewer are working toward a performance activity: one a completed dance and the other a completed interview. Both are connected to some individual or group of individuals communicating through a regular feedback loop. Both work with social context and social boundaries, and both must decide what to include and exclude and what to eventually present in the form of a narrative or story. Another way to look at interviewing is in terms of a creative habit. Like the dancer and choreographer who see dance and its technique as a creative habit, the oral historian as interviewer may view the interview as a creative habit. Many choreographers have written about the creative habit (De Mille, 1992; Hawkins, 1992; Tharp, 2003), as have many social scientists (Csikszentmihalyi, 1996). In my own field of education, it was John Dewey who wrote extensively on this topic (Dewey, 1934). I mention this to point out the cross-disciplinary nature of the idea of habits of mind and body. For the purposes of this book, I focus on interviewing as a creative act dependent on a collection of good habits of mind, as well as practical habits.

INTERVIEWING AS A CREATIVE ACT OF THE IMAGINATION

If we think about the creative act of interviewing, it may be a useful tool for oral historians and other qualitative researchers. Creativity is essentially about discovery, and interviewing allows us a great deal of discovery about a person's life, as well as allowing an understanding of ourselves as researchers. I use the word *creativity* here in the sense in which Csikszentmihalyi (1996) views creativity—as a process by which a symbolic domain in the culture is changed. The creative act of interviewing is such a process, for the symbolic meaning of the interview, its analysis and interpretation, and its final narrative form change the landscape of the historical record. Each researcher, dancer, choreographer, or social scientist is called on to develop habits of mind and body that change the culture. One practical habit for the interviewer might involve preparing materials for the interview—such as testing the digital voice recorder, bringing an extra thumb drive for the recorder, or bringing a battery charger. In other words, all the technical components need to be in order to facilitate the creative habit of interviewing. In addition, being at the site of the interview ahead of time to test equipment and see that the setting is in order is always a good practical habit to develop. Another habit of mind is to compose as many thoughtful questions as possible. It is far better to be overprepared than to get caught in an interview without questions. Usually five or six questions of the type described in the following section are reasonable and may yield well over an hour of interview data on tape. A simple question such as "Tell me about your day as an airline pilot" once yielded nearly 2 hours of interview data, leaving all the other questions for another interview time. You will learn to develop a sense of awareness and timing about your participants in the study and rearrange accordingly. All these habits help to make way for the creative act of interviewing.

Probably the most rewarding component of any qualitative research project is interviewing, because it is a creative act and often requires the use of imagination, much like the choreographer imagining what the dance will look like. In addition to the habits noted earlier, another useful habit to develop before the actual interview is reading recent texts and articles on interviewing (e.g., see Kvale & Brinkmann, 2009; Rubin & Rubin, 2005). Oral history texts and feminist research methods texts also have described interviewing in great detail, including those by Yow (1994, 2005), Reinharz (1992), and Hesse-Biber and Leavy (2007). A good deal of what can be learned about interviewing ultimately may come from trial and error within long-term oral history projects. I have defined interviewing earlier (Janesick, 2004) as a meeting of two persons to exchange information and ideas through questions and responses, resulting in communication and joint construction of meaning about a particular topic. With that in mind, as we are always researchers in the process of conducting a study, we rely on different kinds of questions for eliciting various responses.

ORAL HISTORY INTERVIEWING

Interviewing is an ancient technique, and for the purposes of this book, I define it in this way:

> *Interviewing is a meeting of two persons to exchange*
> *information and ideas through questions and responses,*
> *resulting in communication and joint construction of meaning*
> *about a particular topic.*

Especially in oral history interviews, the participants are focusing on key issues of the past and the present and freely communicate their thoughts through a give-and-take, so to speak, of responses and questions. In two recently completed oral histories of female school superintendents, for example, I had a series of basic questions to start the interviews. The participants, however, had a way of restating and restructuring some of the questions, and we had a dialogue of sorts on the meaning that accompanied the questions. In an earlier work (Janesick, 2004), I described types of questions for qualitative researchers to think about when designing interviews, and I am amending these thoughts here for study.

TYPES OF INTERVIEW QUESTIONS

1. Basic descriptive or "help-me-understand" questions. "Can you talk to me about the recent decision you spoke of earlier which gave you such stress concerning putting students on probation? Tell me what happened following this decision. Help me understand what you meant by the statement 'They are like thorns in my side.'"

2. Structural/paradigmatic questions. "Of all the things you have told me about being a female superintendent, what keeps you going every day? Can you walk me through a typical day? What are some of your proudest achievements?"

3. Follow-up/clarifying questions. "You mentioned that 'face-to-face time with board members' is important to you. Can you tell me how you use this time? Tell me more about what you mean by

your description as a 'techno guru' by those teachers you super-vise."

4. Experience/example questions. "You mentioned that you are seeing students succeed in ways you never imagined. Can you give me an example of this success? Can you give me an example of your most difficult day during your interviews for this position?"

5. Comparison/contrast questions. "You said there was a big dif-ference between a great leader and an ordinary one. What are some of these differences? Can you describe a few for me? You mentioned that there is no simple board meeting and that at the same time you can almost predict what will be the point of contention at the meet-ing. Can you say more about this?"

6. Closing questions. Closing an interview is often difficult for both interviewer and interviewee. Another good rule of thumb for this situation is to ask questions that indicate the end of the inter-view and that also enable the participant to keep thinking about the information already given and quite possibly look forward to another interview. Here are two solid questions for closing an inter-view: "Is there anything you wish to add to our conversation today?" and "Is there anything I have forgotten to ask and which you feel is important?" Notice that there is always room for the participant to elegantly deal with the end of the interview in the moment with such a closing set of questions. In fact, many researchers report that participants will call a day or two later saying they are still thinking about these closing questions and want to tell the researcher some-thing that was forgotten at the time of the interview.

PREPARING QUESTIONS

A good rule of thumb for interviewing is to be prepared—not just with your questions for the interview but also in terms of having all your equipment for interviews in good shape. In order to test some of the questions you create, be sure to do a pilot study of your ques-tions. Find someone to interview, and test the questions. It will save you tons of time later in follow-up interview time. In addition, here are some helpful strategies for success in interviewing.

1. First, **be prepared** with your materials, such as a tape recorder, tape, and a notebook to take field notes while interviewing. Today, digital voice recorders are tremendously economical, efficient, and effective. For less than $90 you can get a digital voice recorder with a thumb drive. This thumb drive can then be attached to your computer and the interview transferred to a CD. Also, the file that is made can be sent electronically to a transcriber. Many of my students have either Olympus or Sony digital recorders, and each year they are upgraded. I myself have had four recorders over the past 4 years, and each is more sophisticated than the last. It is always a good idea to take at least two recorders with you so as to have a backup should one fail you in the field. Likewise, if your recorder uses batteries, be kind to yourself and take extra batteries with you. In Appendix Q of this book, you will find a list of current digital and minicassette recorders that can be purchased online or even at major retailers that sell electronics. Many of my students have decided to use video digital recording, which captures the participant's nonverbal cues, as well as the spoken words. This provides a visual as well as an audio history of a person's story. Digital video cameras are also readily available, ranging from less than $120 to $400. You may purchase a camera that also has appropriate cords for attaching to your TV so that you can see the entire interview on TV. This is often useful at the point of member checking with your participants. Be sure to use technology to your advantage.

2. Before the interview, **check your recorder and/or tape** to see that both are functional. Test your voice on the tape by recording the **DATE, TIME, PLACE,** and **NAME OF THE PARTICIPANT.** This is helpful not only when you do the transcriptions of the tape but also in jarring your memory at a subsequent date. In addition, it helps in coding the data when you are ready to write up your oral history narrative.

3. Whenever possible, **carry a spare tape recorder, extra tapes, and batteries.** Many cases have been described in which the tape was malfunctioning, the recorder died, or the batteries wore out. Weather conditions may also affect your recording apparatus. Be mindful of time as well. Most people cannot sit down for hours at a time for an interview. Try to aim for about an hour of interview time for each of your interviews.

4. If you feel more comfortable giving a copy of the interview questions to your participant, do so ahead of time. This enables the participant to think about the questions in advance and may assist in jogging his or her memory as well as in getting to the heart of the information to be disclosed. You may even find that a participant will change the questions as needed, which is perfectly reasonable and part of this process.

5. Call ahead to remind the participant and to verify the exact date, time, and place of the interview, and arrive early. Remember, in field work anything can happen. In the social world chaos most often reigns. Expect that now and then people will cancel, forget, and reschedule an interview. In rare situations, after an interview a participant may decide that this activity is not for him or her and may drop out of your study. Be prepared with a back-up list of participants if such is the case.

Following are additional helpful ideas as you design the interview portion of your project:

1. Remember the categories of culture that affect how you frame and deliver the question, how you take field notes as the tape is recording, and ultimately how you make sense of the data.

   a. Cognitive culture—how the interviewer and interviewee perceive their own contexts and cultures.

   b. Collective culture—how both see themselves as part of a collective culture, including gender, race, class, religion, and ethnicity.

   c. Descriptive culture—all those written works and works of art and science that have had an effect on both the interviewee and the person who takes the role of interviewer.

2. Be aware of the following assumptions while interviewing someone.

   a. Assumption of similarities. Even though you may professionally act in a role—as, say, an educator interviewing another educator—you should not assume similarity of thoughts, beliefs, values, and so forth.

b. Language difference. The importance of one's own first language and the misinterpretation of meaning in another language is critical.

c. Nonverbal misinterpretation. Obviously we may all read nonverbal language incorrectly; that is the reason that you interview someone more than once.

d. Stereotypes. Before you do any interviewing consider any stereotypes you may hold and be clear about their description in your role as a researcher.

e. Tendency to evaluate. Although most educators continue to evaluate every spoken or written word, even outside the classroom, try to avoid evaluating the content of given remarks.

f. Stress of interviewing. If you are stressed, the person being interviewed may pick up on those cues. Go to the interview prepared, use all your active listening skills, relax, and enjoy the interview.

3. Construct clear, open-ended questions and allow the person to disclose. Avoid interrupting your participants in the study. Avoid leading the witness.

ABOUT PHONE INTERVIEWS

At times, a researcher may need to do a phone interview—in an emergency, to jump-start a project as a preinterview, or to follow up on some information via phone. This technique has many drawbacks, the obvious one being that face-to-face communication is not possible. We live in a time in which we rely on avatars—Facebook accounts with imaginary identities, video games, social network sites, and so forth—and it seems that communication is being relegated to more impersonal forms. If you have to use phone interviews, I would suggest using them in moderation. One good idea for practice is to phone someone you know and interview that person on the topic of your choice.

Be sure to take notes on the phone interview. Overall, student reaction to phone interviews is not as positive as to a face-to-face interview. There is a formal feeling to a phone interview, and consequently a gap exists in the type of data one can retrieve from such an interview. In any event, if you have to do this, be sure to be prepared. Be clear about the purpose of the interview, and leave an opening for the interviewee to add additional information with a question such as, Is there anything else you wish to tell me at this time?

SOME INTERVIEWING RULES OF THUMB
FROM THE INTERVIEWER'S POINT OF VIEW

Individuals who are new to interviews often find it hard to allow the participant/narrator to speak without interruption. Some oral historians in training find silence uncomfortable. No need to fear silence. In fact, silence may help to produce some amazing information. Here are some rules of thumb a group of us came up with in discussing this topic:

1. Be aware of time. Stop when you promised to stop rather than letting an interview go on and on. Do not be afraid to make an appointment for a new time.

2. Let there be silence once in a while. If there is a lull in the interview, perhaps the person is thinking ahead or recalling something.

3. Ask for any papers, documents, or artifacts that have been mentioned in the interview. These data may be used later when you are writing up your narrative.

4. Leave the window open for future contact. Ask if you may return or call back if something isn't clear to you, the interviewer.

5. Always observe common courtesy, standard etiquette, and ethical principles, and thank the interviewee.

In many cases new interviewers offer to take the person out for coffee or lunch. This is an individual preference, but it does make the interview situation more humane and may help to establish rapport, trust, and communication. Feel free to find a mutually agreeable place for interviewing. In terms of ethical considerations, it goes without saying that it would be most problematic to interview someone with whom you have a relationship of evaluator or employer. In other words, the interviewer should not be in a dominant role or a role in which information is extorted. It is sensible to avoid such situations. Of course, written consent must be obtained before the interviews are conducted.

PERENNIAL ETHICAL ISSUES
FOR THE INTERVIEWER

All qualitative interviewers and certainly oral historians face perennial ethical issues as they move from the interview to the writing up of the narrative, and particularly so with oral history. Those of us in public work, such as the field of education, have even more sensitivity to the notion of what it means to work in a public arena. We have to answer to many publics. We have accrediting bodies, federal regulations, state regulations, and of course the institutional review boards (IRBs) watching with a zealous eye. Thus we simply accept the fact that we will always be dealing with ethical issues in all phases of our research. Yes, all researchers work with IRBs, but because of the composition of IRBs and other factors, qualitative research work, particularly oral history, often pays a higher price for its craft. This subject is taken up more fully later in this chapter. For example, one of the most persistent questions for oral historians has to do with using the actual name of the participant. On the one hand, when you document a portion of a life, you want the reader to know whose life it is. On the other hand, in certain situations participants themselves ask that their names be changed in the process of member checking or in the writing-up stage of oral history. The ethical issue concerns confidentiality, anonymity, and quite possibly any resulting damage in the event actual names are identified. What is one to do? I like to err on the side of caution and follow the rule **do no harm**.

If a participant wants a name change to ensure some modicum of safety for any reason, I always agree to change the name. Many of my graduate students have been refused IRB approval because they wished to keep the actual names of the participants in a given study. (This, by the way, was at the request of the participants, who insisted that their names be known.) A good middle way, at least one that my students have agreed to, is to use the letters of the person's actual name to create a pseudonym. For example, the name "Elizabeth Cunningham" can be reformulated as "Beth Chung," both using letters from the person's name and appeasing IRB members who object to actual names. Although this is not a perfect solution, it may be viewed as a good compromise. Of course, it is always advisable to have a good pseudonym handy. For example, if the person's name can suggest the meaning of the person's life, it helps in understanding the narrative. A student of mine who recently studied outstanding female principals chose to name the participants after great historical female leaders to suggest the qualities of each participant—names such as Eleanor Roosevelt, Hillary Clinton, Sojourner Truth, and Margaret Thatcher. The point is that there are ongoing ethical issues that require attention for all oral histories, as well as ethical issues that may arise in each particular oral history.

Recently, for example, the IRB has inserted itself in oral history in a number of ways, only the most obvious of which is the insistence on changing the names of the participants. If you work at an institution that requires IRB approval for oral history projects, then it is wise to fill out the form (see Appendix D) and go through the process. Beginning researchers at the doctoral level who may be conducting their first formal research project are, of course, encouraged to go through the IRB review process. One wonders if it is possible to have complete anonymity in our technological world, designed to avoid privacy. In this very book, I have chosen to use the surnames of well-known choreographers as pseudonyms to protect the participants. We can only do our best to safeguard participants while still staying true to the purposes of oral history. Likewise, as universities become more corporate, the IRB also becomes more corporate. **Oral history has been a field always** *for* **informed consent and always** *for* signed releases and rigor in technique. It is ironic that oral history is the field that has regularly been singled out for so-called IRB transgressions.

IRBs and the Oral Historian: Lessons Learned as a Former IRB Member

Something of a controversy has been brewing in academia since the 1990s about the need for IRB approval in oral history projects. Key professional organizations, such as the Oral History Association and the American Historical Association, have been active in pursuing exclusion of oral history from the IRB process. In a nutshell, the controversy comes down to this. On the one hand, we want to protect all participants by getting IRB approval for any research, including oral history research. On the other hand, the federal regulations indicate that IRB approval is not needed for oral history, basically because it is not scientific enough in terms of generalizability and hypothesis testing. In 2004, federal guidelines totally exempted oral history from the IRB process; since then things have been changing, depending on which universities involve themselves in such cases. For a complete update on these matters, it is helpful to visit the sites of the Oral History Association (OHA; *alpha.dickinson.edu/oha/org_irb.html*) and of the American Historical Association (AHA; *www.historians.org/perspectives/issues/2008/0802/0802aha1.cfm*) (see Appendices F and G for detailed statements). Consequently, I have become increasingly interested in the problems arising for qualitative researchers, particularly doctoral students doing oral history, when the IRB forms are open for review and approval.

As a qualitative researcher all my life, an oral historian in the past two decades, and a recent member of an IRB at a previous institution, I am able to look back on the lessons learned from these experiences. I was an active IRB member for a 3-year term and was the only qualitative researcher, let alone oral historian, of 11 members. The university was in a metropolitan area and had a student population of around 7,000 students. At the time there were only two doctorates offered at the university: Doctor of Education (EdD) and Doctor of Psychology (PsyD). The workload was steady, and there was one IRB. By contrast, at my current institution, there are 45,000 students and five IRBs, four for medicine and one for all other studies, particularly the social sciences and humanities. At the time of my service on the board, I was, coincidentally, the program director of a doctoral program in the College of Education. My students were directly affected on a daily basis. The types of questions asked of qualitative researchers by IRB members, the ethical issues raised by these questions, and the burden put on the shoulders of the researchers involved had raised my interest to the point of writing about this. Here I describe and explain three cases based on the lived experience of my students to illuminate strategies for dealing with the IRB.

CASE II.1.
☙

The Researcher-and-Participant Relationship

This case draws on the experience of individual graduate students who were studying practitioners in public and private schools, as well as other community venues. They were interviewing participants for oral histories, observing them, and keeping a researcher's reflective journal. They also asked their participants to write reflective journals as well. In addition, one doctoral student did an interactive journal with the participants. In trying to capture this on the IRB form, all researchers were direct, descriptive, and forthright. Unfortunately, all applications were returned with similar questions. As a result, the students were prevented from moving on in the process for periods of between 1 and 6 months and, in one case, even longer. Nonetheless, all students followed the suggestions of the IRB to gain approval and complete the dissertation research.

One of the goals of the IRB is to "meet regularly" and have a "timely turnaround" with a decision to enable students to proceed with their work. Although all IRBs exist and thrive in local campus cultures and with local hierarchies of power, it is helpful to learn from the actual experience of the cases to follow. These cases present samples of the questions and comments returned to the prospective researchers with few suggestions or alternatives, but to which students deftly and purposefully replied. All the students were female professionals with many years of experience in educational leadership at all levels of work, elementary through university. They were persistent with e-mails and phone calls to IRB members and in face-to-face meetings with them. These examples are summaries of the more lengthy dialogues that took place. They are related here to serve as learning examples for prospective qualitative researchers as they begin to deal with IRBs. In each case, the approval of the project was held up until the researcher responded in writing and resubmitted the form a second or third time. It was astounding to students who had in good faith produced all the correct forms and wanted just to proceed with their research projects.

IRB MEMBER STATEMENT: Why keep a journal? These are too personal.

RESEARCHER RESPONSE: The researcher presented the IRB member with a three-page bibliography of the books, articles, and book chapters on this very topic. The basic argument presented was that the history of journal writing goes back in the arts and sciences for centuries. In this case the researcher used a historical argument to win over the IRB member. In addition, the researcher argued that the confidentiality and anonymity agreement between all persons involved in this project protected all of us, including the university. The researcher also used a type of legal argument by finding one legal case that supported her position. Faced with the evidence, the IRB member then voted to approve the project. This seemed to work. Note that if even one IRB member raises questions, the entire process may be stalled.

IRB MEMBER: Who is going to read these journals?

RESEARCHER RESPONSE: The researcher politely asked the board member to see a particular page X, on which it was stated that only this researcher and these participants will read these journals. Once again, the researcher brought the written evidence to the meeting to remind the member that, in fact, this was clearly stated in the proposal. In order to get her proposal passed, the researcher agreed to use, in the appendices of her dissertation, one example from the reflective journal that related only to her own recollections of the research process she constructed. This was the only option for her at the time to gain approval, and she wanted to move on and finish. It appeared that the snag involved any data in a journal from the participant in the study.

IRB MEMBER: Are your interview questions tested? (This was within the context of a proposal that clearly described the pilot study with its pilot interview and questions.)

RESEARCHER RESPONSE: The student politely pointed to the proposal statement about testing the questions in a pilot study. Again, the researcher was amazingly persistent in tracking down the IRB member and intractably persuasive regarding the exact pages and exact lines of the evidence in the proposal. She even went so far as to ask the member whether perhaps he was thinking of another proposal rather than her proposal. One major headache that surfaced at this time was how to track down an IRB member. Some professors arrived on campus only a few minutes before their class time and at no other time. It was up to the doctoral student to find the person and gain a satisfactory response to be able to even get to the resubmittal stage of the project.

IRB MEMBER: How can you have a co-researcher in a project?

RESEARCHER RESPONSE: The student here, with kindness and respect, pointed out that it is surely possible to have a co-researcher relationship in the field. She stated that in her field, educational leadership, this has been done before. The researcher provided a bibliography to help on this point. In addition, the researcher was savvy enough to know that she had to find an example in the field of this IRB member, a psychologist, and she found one rather effortlessly. She inquired into the names of current doctoral students in psychology, and she was able to find three examples in recent dissertations in that department. Nonetheless, the IRB member then requested of the applicant that she find an article, a book, and any other evidence for this member before he would sign off on it. She found it. He approved it.

IRB MEMBER: It is unethical to observe people. (He thought she was not informing the participants of the observation.)

RESEARCHER RESPONSE: The researcher replied that there is a long and elegant history of observation, description, and explanation that is the cornerstone of all good science and research. In fact, she provided examples of definitions from various dictionaries of the word *empirical*, including "direct observation of experience," "experience," and "real-world experience." She also provided additional evidence with an annotated bibliography that detailed books on qualitative research methods, along with some sample illustrative studies that successfully incorporated observations and interviews, similar to the proposed study.

IRB MEMBER: I do not think this university is one that is interested in your type of research or research topic.

RESEARCHER RESPONSE: Here again the researcher respectfully disagreed on this point. She thought the university would be proud of the study, which documented how two former gang members actually returned to school to get their high school diplomas through an equivalency program. As a professional who worked with and studied gang behavior, she suggested that the study might inspire others to return and complete their educations. In addition, she pointed out that she had followed all the guidelines set forth by the government and by the university. She found, in writing, the regulations and provided them on the spot. Still the IRB member would not be satisfied. The student made numerous attempts to bombard this IRB member with written information regarding the educational interest and value of studying former gang members, yet it was quite some time before she wore down this individual and finally won approval.

IRB MEMBER: How will you replicate and generalize your case study?

RESEARCHER RESPONSE: The student reiterated the value of case study research and oral history, which are widely used in many of the social sciences, the medical professions, and the arts and humanities. "The value is that the case teaches us something. The case is unique. We can never set up exact and duplicative cases. This is not suitable for generalizing. The study is designed to help me and others learn from this case." She was also proactive and provided a list of resources on the method. The student also provided the board member with six textbooks on exemplary case studies and a list of case studies in dissertation abstracts; this seemed to be the best strategy at the time. She was determined to triumph, and she eventually did so.

IRB MEMBER: I do not like your consent form.

RESEARCHER RESPONSE: The student said: "Please help me out here. Please show me what you do not like about the form. It is designed to touch upon all the issues related to consent. I really tried to comply with all the federal guidelines and university guidelines. Can you be specific?" The IRB member objected to the phrase "no harm will come to me." After phone calls, e-mails, and two meetings with the IRB member, the researcher changed the terms as follows: "I, (the participant), understand the purpose of the study and willingly take part in the study." (By the way, the word *harm* is used in the federal guidelines.) The researcher merely changed phrases to accommodate the member's request. She also argued that the federal guidelines themselves, when referring to harm, are taken in a global sense—that is, the guideline for defining "harm" in any research project is the amount or chance of potential harm one might suffer during any everyday activities. The researcher changed the form to include the point that harm should be no more than what one might suffer in ordinary life.

IRB MEMBER: How do you know you are not harming people by interviewing them?

RESEARCHER RESPONSE: Here the IRB member allowed the consent form with the words "no harm will come to me." However, the member was concerned about interviewing as a research technique. The doctoral student responded in this way: "As you can see, my questions provided in the application, Interview Protocol A, are designed to gain information about a school leader's views on her work. Let's take a look at these questions and, as we do so, can you tell me which you think are harmful?" The questions were:

- Describe for me your typical day as the principal of this school.
- Can you talk to me about your single most noteworthy achievement?
- Can you think back over this past year and describe a situation which caused you to seek outside help on any matter?
- Can you talk about a situation where you struggled and struggled over a solution to a problem at the time, yet now months later, can only laugh about it?

The student continued, "I can assure you that I am asking these questions of a remarkably sophisticated and articulate professional to help me to achieve the goals of my study. In no way are these intended to be harmful in any way." This approach seemed to work.

IRB MEMBER: I will not approve this study unless you change your consent form to say that this dissertation will appear in *Dissertation*

Abstracts [a central international database] and that this study may be read by someone in the future. After all, you are using interviews and journals.

RESEARCHER RESPONSE: The courteous researcher asked, "Are not all studies on *Dissertation Abstracts*, whether they use qualitative methods or quantitative methods? Since I said in my form this was my dissertation study, does that not suffice?" In order to proceed and to assuage the IRB member, the researcher added the wording about the dissertation appearing in *Dissertation Abstracts* after much soul-searching and at least three face-to-face meetings with the member who was holding up the process. The student eventually wrote about the angst involved in this process as an ethical component of field-work in her final chapter of her dissertation. Still, the student viewed this conflict as a personal issue. She felt her only alternative was to meet the demand of the IRB member for fear of losing even more time. She "complied under duress," as she put it.

You can see, even with this small number of instances, the numerous questions posed to oral historians and qualitative researchers. The process of responding to questions posed by IRB members made it clear that some members:

1. Had little or no knowledge of the procedures, theory, history, or work of qualitative researchers in general and oral historians in particular and, in fact, waited for responses from applicants to provide evidence regarding methods.

2. Were requiring a standard for qualitative researchers unlike that of other researchers, for example, requiring additional statements not required by the federal guidelines and not required of those using quantitative methods.

3. Had never thought about including qualitative researchers, let alone oral historians, on the board itself. The only reason I became a member of the IRB was that I raised the issue of the extensive questioning of qualitative researchers being disproportionate to the entire applicant pool with my then provost. The provost, who appoints members to the IRB, said to me, "You are now a member

of the IRB, effective immediately, and the paperwork will follow today."

4. Imposed upon qualitative researchers norms used in experimental and quasi-experimental projects from fields unlike education, history, and other professions.

5. Viewed proposals against one standard that disavowed both the idea of co-researchers in a project and the possibility of multiple and alternative methods of research (see also Shea, 2000).

Following a discussion of these points, I argue for the need for qualitative researchers and oral historians to **adopt strategies of actions** that respond to the following questions:

- How can oral historians and other qualitative researchers be proactive in addressing and foreseeing the eventual questions asked by IRB members who may not know of the history, practice, and literature in our field?
- How can we be proactive and gain IRB membership?
- How can we do a better job in explaining what IRB members do?

Lessons Learned from This Case

As you can see, just the types of questions sent back to the prospective researchers are quite revealing. In many instances they show a surprising absence of understanding about the nature of oral history. Some may even say there is a bias against history in some cases. Doctoral students expressed disappointment at the way they were treated. Particularly surprising was the resistance to interviewing or journal writing or any technique that was focused on personal meaning. Luckily, each of the students was persistent in responding to the questions posed and used direct citations with evidence from current research methodology texts. In addition, doctoral students had to make numerous phone calls, send numerous e-mails, and personally try to track down IRB members to speak on behalf of their applications for approval. They were well prepared for this after the initial written queries by the IRB members. They became activists for their research. As a sort of soothing balm, many of the students wrote about these efforts in their individual dissertations—under the topic of ethical issues and fieldwork—or in subsequent written work. Others just changed their methods to use generic case studies, which seemed to work in terms of gaining IRB approval. Students who were going on to be the next generation of researchers and professors swore that they would be extremely vigilant in terms of their own students and interactions with future IRB members. They also expressed a deep sense of perplexity over what we might be losing as a field when we deny the value of oral history.

CASE II.2.

The Qualitative Researcher and Representations of Data

Although numerous books and articles exist on representation of data in qualitative studies, I wish to focus on one case of a student who was denied IRB approval on the basis of a request by participants in the study. Participants requested that the researcher use their real names rather than pseudonyms. In this case, the individual names had significance to the participants and to the researcher in terms of how the data were to be represented. This issue itself caused a 6-month delay in approval for the student. The IRB member and the student went back and forth on this. I was a member of the student's committee, so I was excused from the deliberation, as was the practice for IRB members. None of us read applications from our own students. I did ask the student what she would like to do, and she said she wanted to move on and get approval. So I made the suggestion discussed earlier in hopes of satisfying all parties: Take the letters of the names in question and change them into other names, attempting to use as many of the original letters as possible. Thus you still retain something of the person's name in that the same letters are used. For example, the name "Miranda Steele" can become the pseudonym "Diana Lester." The student played around with this idea, checked with the members, and more or less reached agreement. The IRB was satisfied that original names were not used. The student was happy to move on. The participants were perplexed by the consternation over such a simple request to use their own names. This solution, though imperfect, seemed to work at the time and permitted the student to proceed.

What was raised for discussion afterward, under the aegis of representation of data and ethical concerns in qualitative research projects, was that this most personal of identifiers, one's own name, was a point of contention. Qualitative work in general and most certainly oral history seek to tell someone's personal, lived experience and what it means. Ironically, **this case resulted in erasure of the individuals' actual names.** This moved the discussion to purposes of the IRB, which originally emerged from the biomedical model. The IRB was intended to protect the persons in any given study. Currently it appears that the focus has turned to fear of lawsuits as the motivating force. Is it not time to continue and enlarge the discussion on the goals, focus, parameters, and purposes of IRBs in social science research? And can we not rediscover the original intent of the IRB? Have we not the creativity and imagination to deal with framing the discourse beyond the legal concerns? Currently, many journals in the social sciences, pharmacology, education, nursing, the humanities, and medicine are in fact raising some of these powerful questions. In addition, there are numerous blogs on IRB issues related to oral historians. In fact, some universities work out ways in which, in specific cases of oral history, they do not come totally under IRB jurisdiction. To date there are five such universities. I discuss this issue more fully later in this book in the context of ethical and legal issues in oral history.

CASE II.3.
༺

The Qualitative Researcher as Co-Researcher with Participants in a Project

The doctoral student who decided to list her participants as co-researchers really got a surprise when her application was stopped cold. She used e-mail, phone, and face-to-face meetings to try to persuade the board member. No agreement could be reached, so she decided to move on and list the participants as participants. The life energy she was using was too much of a loss. She decided that she would write an article at a date well after the final defense of the dissertation in which she would use the concept of co-researcher as a central piece. This case calls to mind the argument so beautifully captured by Lincoln and Tierney (2004). Basically, they have argued that, although it is not necessarily intentional, many IRBs basically use blocking behavior rather than facilitating behavior in dealing with qualitative research proposals in general. The result then ends up rather chaotic. Projects are often sidelined and are required to go through multiple revisions, as in the cases previously mentioned. They also described five critical conclusions based on similar stories from other researchers related to the IRB interaction. They pointed out the following serious repercussions.

1. Widespread rejection of qualitative research projects suggest that these **findings will be heard less in policy forums**, if at all.

2. Qualitative researchers are taking on the responsibility for confronting the control of discourse by traditional elites.

3. New researchers and scholars trained in alternative methods find their inquiries rejected.

4. Government documents show that the actual definition of research is a narrow one despite all scholarship to the contrary.

5. This resistance and rejection suggests that traditional elites actually do understand the power of strong qualitative studies, which are data rich and are valid (Lincoln & Tierney, 2004, pp. 231–232).

I mention all this to alert the reader to the ongoing tension, discourse, and practice relative to IRB issues and the oral historian. We need to talk through this state of affairs. Professional meetings are one way to raise the level of interest and discourse on these matters. Another means available is writing. Notable journals in various person-oriented fields are dedicating entire journals to these topics of ethical issues and the IRB. For example, nearly an entire issue of the journal *Qualitative Inquiry* (Vol. 10, No. 2, April 2004) was devoted to substantive questions and issues related to IRBs and qualitative research. In fact, in many of the disciplines mentioned earlier, entire conferences, journals, and discussion boards have been devoted to similar discussions of the IRB and qualitative researchers. In addition, many journals in the fields of history, sociology, ethics, Internet inquiry and online journals have addressed these and other related questions. By the time this book is in print, ongoing and additional blogs, newsletters, and journals of professional organizations such as the Oral History Association (OHA) may also have treated these topics more deeply. Some have already suggested that we approach the IRB by recasting our work as an innovation.

About Approaching IRBs as an Innovation

The recent literature on innovations suggests that innovations can succeed when all parties involved learn the language involved, get on board and develop an open mind toward the innovation, and, in fact, gain membership in the process itself. Although qualitative research has an ancient and firm pedigree and, in fact, is older than statistical methods, to recast our work as an innovation may help to persuade traditional elites about the meaning, value, and power of qualitative research projects. I found it helpful to stress the long and eloquent history of qualitative research and to back that up with a data list of references and resources. In addition, the argument for treating oral history as an innovation within the context of the history of the IRB makes sense. The famous Belmont Report, issued in 1978, was the eventual code adopted for research guidelines for the IRB regarding human participants. The basic ethical guidelines set forth by the Belmont Report included **respect for persons, beneficence, and justice**. *Respect for persons* included support for human dignity and informed consent. *Beneficence* involves protection from harm and minimal risks in research. *Justice* requires benefits and burdens to be fairly distributed. At the time and in the report, research was defined as hypothesis testing and generalizability as its result. Obviously this has the potential of creating problems for oral history and any other form of qualitative research approach. I found that many IRB members were swayed a tiny bit by references on the Web. In that spirit, here are some resources readily available on the Web. These are a few sites that many doctoral students and some IRB members have found helpful.

WEB RESOURCES FOR QUALITATIVE RESEARCHERS AND IRBs

www.irb.pitt.edu. At this site, see the IRB e-mail archives with such topics as (1) Ask the IRB, (2) Research Practice Fundamentals, and (3) Research Involving Children.

www.copernicusgroup.com. See this site for information such as (1) the Belmont Report, (2) a medical glossary, and (3) applied ethics from ARENA (Applied Research Ethics National Association), an organization that deals with ethical practice, regulations, and policy regarding research and clinical practice.

www.hhs.gov/ohrp. This site provides information about recent cases, as well as providing links to Web resources on human-subjects research.

www.hhs.gov/ohrp. See this site—from the Office for Human Research Protections, U.S. Department of Health and Human Services—for policy guidance, educational materials, compliance oversight, and workshops.

www.irbforum.org. The Institutional Review Board—Discussion and News Forum (IRB Forum) promotes discussion on ethics, regulations, problems, and policy regarding human subjects.

SELECTED ARTICLES FROM JOURNALS THAT REGULARLY FOCUS ON IRB ISSUES

Evaluation Review

Oakes, J. M. (2002). Risks and wrongs in social science research: An evaluator's guide to the IRB. Vol. 26, No. 5, pp. 443–479.

Ethics and Behavior

Gunsalus, C. K. (2004). The nanny state meets the inner lawyer: Over-regulating while protecting human participants in research. Vol. 14, No. 4, pp. 369–382.

Western Journal of Nursing Research

Frewda, M. C., & Kearney, M. H. (2005). Ethical issues faced by nursing editors. Vol. 27, No. 4, pp. 487–499.

Spotlight on Research

Kim, E. (2004, July/August). Protection of child human subjects. pp. 161–167.

Academic Medicine

Tomkowiak, J. M., & Gunderson, A. J. (2004). To IRB or not to IRB? Vol. 79, No. 7, pp. 628–632.

Kennedy Institute of Ethics Journal

Holt, E. (2002). Expanding human research oversight. Vol. 12, No. 2, pp. 215–224.

These journals and sample articles capture some of the current discussion, but this is not meant to be an exhaustive list.

All in all, the Web is a good source for up-to-the-minute discussions, blogs, policy changes, and guidelines that may be of some assistance to researchers. In checking on the Web recently by simply typing the letters "IRB" into *www.hhs.gov/ohrp/irb/irb*, I found more than 122,000 references and websites. You will find numerous weblogs (blogs), university sites with helpful cases, and policies and extensive interpretations of the federal guidelines. Other resources can be found in journals, most often in education, the humanities, medicine, pharmacy, and social work. Likewise the IRB blog *www.institutionalreviewblog.com* is an outstanding resource. In reviewing many of the websites, I found a cluster of issues noted that include but are not limited to the following and that merit further study:

1. Questions about the ethics of studying, interviewing, and even observing children. Some of those questions revolve around issues of informed consent, children's ability to answer questions without fear of judgment or dislike, and children's rights.

2. Anonymity, namely, how anonymous is anonymous? For example, with a good description of persons, places, events, and location of the university at which the dissertation is completed, can

it be that difficult to identify which institution, which persons, and which sites are studied?

3. Confidentiality related to the techniques of journal writing.

4. Whether action research, particularly participatory action research, teacher research, and classroom research, is nonscientific.

5. Moving our various fields forward and widening the repertoire of research techniques.

6. The question of who research is for in the end. Is it for the researcher? Is it for changing the world?

7. Policy implications and discussions that qualitative researchers are excluded from systematically and otherwise.

Practical Strategies for the Steps to Success

As I often tell my students and colleagues, always expect the unexpected when dealing with the IRB if your project is qualitative. The issues raised on this topic will not go away. In fact, as more and more students stand up to rejection notices from their IRB member(s), discussions will only escalate. Many already have framed these issues in the larger context of institutional and bureaucratic lethargy. I have found the following strategies helpful in addressing the conflict and tension raised by rejecting scholarly proposals, and I recommend the following:

1. Request membership on the IRB.

2. Prepare a selected bibliography supporting your study to hand to the IRB member if the proposal is rejected. Even more effective is to meet with the member and bring a few current methods texts.

3. Take the IRB member out for coffee or lunch to explain informally what you will follow up with formally.

4. Get a selected and appropriate list of completed dissertations in your field that are listed on the Pro Quest site *www.proquest.com* and that used alternative qualitative methods over the past 15 years or so.

5. In all research courses include a module on dealing with the IRB, as well as the history, purposes, conflicts, and written statutes regarding the IRB. There are many excellent articles in print and on the Web.

6. Take some time to learn the language of the traditionalist.

7. Avoid caving in. Persistence is critical.

8. In your university, encourage multiple IRB panels, as many universities already have. For example, at my current institution we have six IRB panels. Five of these are constructed for the medical school, and one is designed for all other social science research projects. A strong case can be made for including qualitative researchers, especially oral historians, on the social science IRB.

9. Open the conversation about these issues at your own university to begin a dialogue on the topic. Use the various examples from resources mentioned here and elsewhere. Become an agent of change at your site.

What have I learned as a member of the IRB? Among other things, I have learned that ethics has been relegated to the area of informed consent. Regularly, the IRB institutional forms seem to be designed to avoid lawsuits. At some future date, someone might think about writing on this topic and rewriting IRB forms. I have also learned how important it is to educate professionals on the IRB. You would be surprised at how a reading list can make a world of difference. Something as simple as a list of current texts and reports on qualitative research methods can keep many a member of the IRB supportive. To close this section with a reflection on the metaphor of dance, these strategies for effective communication between qualitative researchers and IRB members are similar to the work of the choreographer. Isn't it more productive for all of us to get on with the dance? Can we all try out the steps together? Can we work to have equal representation on IRBs? The nuts-and-bolts IRB form itself is born of a modernist medical-model perspective, and qualitative research projects often are postmodern if not beyond. Qualitative researchers need to be sophisticated enough to manage to describe their proposed projects in the modernist idiom without sacrificing

the story and its participants. Oral historians and other qualitative researchers need to redefine the choreography of matriculating
through the IRB process, as every generation of dancers in dance
history has refined choreography throughout the ages. We live in an
exciting time, for we have the opportunity and power to do this.

ANALYZING AND INTERPRETING ORAL HISTORY INTERVIEW DATA

With awareness of some of the techniques of interviewing, as well
as of potential ethical issues involved with oral history interviewing,
the demanding task of analyzing interview data and making sense
of it begins. A good rule of thumb upon completing an interview is
to transcribe it as soon as possible. There are many transcription
services available on the Web in the event that you are unable to
do your own transcriptions. To give just two examples, Production
Transcripts in Los Angeles (*www.productiontranscripts.com*) is one
of the most active. Another website is *www.castingwords.com*; many
have found it effective and efficient in terms of turnaround time and
content. With the transcripts in hand, the researcher may read and
reread them as the process of analysis and interpretation begins.
Researchers look for major themes, key words, and indices of behavior and belief and make an initial list of major and minor categories.
Every attempt is made to look for critical incidents, points of tension and conflict, and contradictions to help in interpreting the data.
See the following example of a written narrative of an individual's
account of her work and her growth as a professional, which can be
viewed as a feminist account of this portion of her life.

As Reinharz (1992) demonstrated in Chapter 7 of *Feminist Methods in Social Research*, "women's oral history . . . is a feminist encounter even if the interviewee is not herself a feminist" (p. 126). This
particular chapter, titled "Feminist Oral History," is helpful in framing oral history as part of a social justice project by virtue of helping
the reader understand how biographical work such as oral history
takes women out of obscurity, repairs the historical record, and provides an opportunity for the woman reader and writer to identify

with the lived experience of the person participating in the interview (Reinharz, 1992, pp. 126–144). Consider the following excerpt as such an example.

CASE II.4.
ༀ

An Oral History Co-Constructed Narrative

Assisting Others, Inspiring Self: Reflections of an Educator—
The Story of Lynn T. Tharp, Part of a Response to the Instruction
"Describe Yourself and Your Work."

One of the benefits of living in a large, urban city like Chicago is the cultural diversity that envelops the city. The Art Institute of Chicago was graced with the Seurat exhibit this summer, which I was fortunate to see. Gazing at the paintings caused me to reflect upon the concept of pointillism. It is fascinating to imagine how the artist created a piece based on thousands of tiny dots. In a minute sense, Seurat's work made me think of my own career choice—that of serving as an assistant professor of English and Communications. For me, the decision to pursue a career in higher education was not one event or great epiphany. Rather, it is composed of a series of events and decisions that culminated into the decision. Much like the viewer looking at *A Sunday Afternoon on the Island of La Grande Jatte*, there lie many dots in a span of time that result in a beautiful piece of art, or in my case, a career decision.

For as long as I can remember, my house was filled with books. My grandfather worked as a bookbinder for Rand McNally and my father was a manager of publications and communications, resulting in the creation of a literacy-rich home. Some of my favorite childhood presents were children's classical literature and poem books. Many of these books were given to me by my aunt, who would sit and read to me for hours during those family gatherings.

This early exposure to reading transformed into positive grade school years. I later attended a college-prep high school, which was highly competitive, for the college bound. It wasn't a question of whether or not I would attend college; it was a matter of being accepted into a school that would match my interests and needs, as well as credentials.

I always had an interest in English and journalism in high school and was plagued by math anxiety. Deciding on a major in undergraduate school was difficult. Majoring in English was out of the question because I had no interest in being a teacher. The thought of being a teacher brought to mind visions of ancient, scrawny women and old nuns who seemed to have no life outside of the classroom. Advice for my first major in college came from my father, who said, "The important thing to remember is that it doesn't necessarily matter what your major is in college. It is far greater to pursue a career that is meaningful to you."

While that is sound advice, it was far too esoteric for a freshman. Business was selected as my first major, which lasted 1 year. The math requirement was far too great, and my grade on the freshman math class was definitely not dean's list material. Again, advice was given, although this time much harsher: Change your major or attend a junior college. English and dance were my only two strong points, so I changed my major to political science. It wasn't until my junior year that I realized I could pursue a career in other venues besides teaching, so I graduated with a bachelor of arts in English.

The montage of colors on canvas would not be complete without discussing leadership opportunities experienced in college. Although it was against my rebellious nature at the time, I went through sorority rush my freshman year and obtained a bid from the house of my choice. Although there is a negative stigma about sorority Greeks, there is often little talk about the positive campus and community involvement. My suite mate, who was involved in activities both within the house as well as on campus, offered this piece of advice: "Get involved as much as you can."

Obsessively, I took these words of wisdom to heart. My list of campus activities included: administrative assistant for my house, Pan-Hellenic Vice President, minutes secretary for the Student Association Senate, BACCHUS (Boost Alcohol Conscientiousness Concerning the Health of University Students) president, student health educator, and secretary for Sigma Tau Delta (English Honor Society). Through these activities I had the opportunity to attend and speak at national conferences, attend leadership seminars, and educate others. I received several leadership awards, such as Student and Senior Leader, Order of Omega, Outstanding Greek, and an Institutional Scholarship for Student Leadership.

Another valuable concept I learned during my undergraduate years was the difference between work and a career. During my freshman and sophomore years, I worked in a factory assembling police lights. To this day, I do not know which is more arduous: performing tasks that were physically exhausting or those that were mentally exhausting (i.e., boredom from performing mindless repetitive tasks). The full-time factory workers inspired me in a profound way. Many were women, single supporters of their family, and received no education beyond a high school diploma. Day after day they never complained but dreamed about a better life for their child. I realized that they would never leave the factory; their dreams lay in the hope for a better tomorrow for their children. The factory job was not a career for these women, only a means for survival. I considered myself fortunate to be going to college and vowed that someday I would find a meaningful career.

Life as a summer factory worker ended my junior year as I obtained a summer internship at a publishing company. During the course of two summers, I worked in human resources and learned many aspects of the publishing field. This proved to be valuable experience, as I was offered a full-time job as an editorial assistant after graduation. Within 9 months I was promoted to a developmental editor for accounting textbooks. During this time, I also went back to school to earn a master of arts degree in communications.

Although I very much enjoyed my work in publishing, something was missing. During the course of about 5 years, I worked in various positions in the publishing area, such as an assistant managing editor for a medical publisher and a writer for an employee benefits magazine. After glancing through the job ads, I spied an ad for a part-time ESL [English as a second language] instructor at a local community college. I applied for the position on a Thursday and was in the classroom the following Monday.

Teaching part time opened entirely new doors for me. Long gone were the thoughts of the bitter grammar school teachers. Teaching for me was inspiring and invigorating. Despite working a 40-hour-a-week job, I was energized teaching from 6:00 P.M. until 10:00 P.M. 2 days a week. The first two courses I taught were ESL writing and freshman composition. During this time in political history, the U.S. was experiencing a wave of immigrants from countries such as Haiti and Vietnam. Stories about heroic escapes from homelands and journeys across thousands of miles by boat were displayed in the media. What touched me the most was the fact that these "boat people" were my students. Essays written by these students were filled with tales about hope for a better life in America. On more than one occasion, tears rolled down my cheek as I read their stories of inspiration. From this early teaching experience, I made it my personal mission to gain further teaching experience with the hopes of landing a full-time position in higher education. Finally, I had found my passion.

I continued traditional in-class teaching for City Colleges [in Chicago] before finding a new interest—online teaching. Quality education, in my opinion, could be delivered in an online setting with the right course content design and enthusiasm for teaching. Additionally, online courses provide an opportunity for many students to obtain a college degree. These nontraditional students typically juggle the demands of work, family, and/or physical limitations that make attending class in a traditional way impossible. To this day I continue to teach part time in an online environment.

After submission of many resumes, I finally obtained a position as the Higher Education Basics Director and Assessment Director at a small, private urban college. The demographics of the student population are typically first-generation, minority college students. In my role, I was responsible for overseeing developmental reading, writing, and math courses. Placements for students in this program were [based on] low scores on the college's entrance exam. Thus, the students needed to complete the basics program before matriculating into the regular college curriculum.

My early experiences as a full-time instructor were very Pollyanna, as I believed that all students wanted to earn a college degree, obtain a fulfilling career, and change their lives. It was very disappointing to realize that many students lack the desire to graduate from college. However, it was inspiring to know that an effective instructor has the ability to inspire others and help the dedicated to achieve their dream. During my first year teaching full time I also gave birth to my daughter. I continued working full time until I made the decision to return to school to pursue a doctoral degree in educational leadership and organizational change.

During my doctoral studies I had the opportunity to gain firsthand experience with working with the elementary schools. I designed, managed, and obtained funding for a parent–child literacy program that involved working with a probationary school on Chicago's South Side. It was a real eye-opener to experience the struggles of many lower-income families. Despite heroic efforts by the school administration and staff, there is no way to control the environment a child is raised in. A few blocks outside the "safe school zone" revealed urban warfare and tales of children being shuffled from one caregiver to the next. However, working with the program allowed me to assist parents and children, and one small hug from a child or word of thanks from a parent speak volumes.

Fortunately I was able to identify a career I have true passion for: higher education. With this determination I set forth on my journey. Rough and rocky roads crossed my path. It was extremely difficult raising an 18-month-old little girl almost single-handedly (my husband at the time worked in the nightclub business and was rarely home), studying and attending classes, and working three or four part-time jobs in higher education. However, my passion and determination for completion never waned. Despite personal problems, I was the first in my cohort to successfully defend my dissertation.

I wrote every day, and despite handling many responsibilities, I became consumed with my writing. The demands of a qualitative dissertation are intense, and I often wondered where I drew my inner strength to persevere. After perusing through my reflective journal kept while writing the dissertation, I came across the following entry, the first written in a daily ritual:

September, 2001
After recently hearing a speech from a recent graduate, I felt a wake-up call to the enormous task ahead. However, organization and commitment will get you through. . . . I think my major roadblock is deciding on a topic. Once my focus is clear, the live-breath dissertation process begins. The classroom presentation re-emphasized the importance of organization, dedication, and self-discipline needed to finish the dissertation. Fortunately, I still follow the advice I received in a class taken the first quarter: Do something every day. That's critical, involves sacrifice, but keeps you on top of things.

I realized that qualitative research would get to stories of real people. I also enjoy the interviewing process and learning about others' life experience. So the process, though it involves much more work than crunching numbers from a random survey, seems enjoyable.

In a first attempt to begin the dissertation process, I "cleaned house" and organized old research papers, notes, books, and cleared out file cabinets. I also reread parts of various texts which makes so much more sense to me now than the first read. Although I knew I had anxiety about the dissertation, the chapter helped me recognize these thoughts are completely normal. Most importantly, self-confidence is so, so important. Now is not the time to question writing ability or dedication. Focus and confidence are needed. So, at the present, I have a long way to go in this saga. I truly enjoy writing and researching so once I begin, I will not stop. There is so much I need to learn about qualitative research. The rest lies in my hands. . . . LLT

Completing the dissertation was, by far, the single greatest challenge I have ever faced. Even on the day of the final defense, no break was given to me. Ten days prior I had "minor" surgery that was performed without any problems. The morning of my final defense I awoke, startled to be covered in a pool of blood. I phoned the doctor and told him I would be in the office to see him at 1:00 P.M. Crazed with the thought of delaying the final defense, I focused on the task, defended my dissertation successfully, and later ended up in the E.R.

Perhaps the impact the study had on me can best be expressed from an excerpt from my dissertation:

> As a result of this study, I have grown in knowledge and understanding of not only instructional technology, but also the leadership needed to bring about institutional and departmental changes. For me, I have changed my perspective on the roles of educational leaders and technology use. Prior to this study, I was unaware of the varied nature and responsibilities held by the educational leaders of various levels. I discovered that deans have a genuine interest in student and curriculum concerns. I have also gained a better understanding of the process of change, in particular the steps and challenges involved with incorporating instructional technology use into the curriculum. Through interviewing, observing, and "living" the experiences of the six educational leaders, I was given a unique opportunity to experience their daily activities. It was also an amazing opportunity to learn from their experience. This insight is invaluable as I begin the journey toward pursuing a career in academia.

I have also realized the importance of collaboration, motivation, and teamwork. After reading my journal entries, these elements clearly stood out. Bringing about major changes requires the feedback and advice from everyone in the learning community. Journal writing in itself was an opportunity to reflect on many personal issues. I was able to slow down and reflect upon my experiences during the entire dissertation process. This caused me to analyze the past, live in the present, and plan for the future. I also realized that throughout this process I have grown in ways often difficult to express to others. Journaling provided an outlet for all of the thoughts going on in my head and an opportunity to go back and reflect on the dissertation process and on myself.

This study also enabled me to focus on a future career path. I have always enjoyed technology and learning about ways it can improve my life. It was enjoyable talking to others about their experiences with technology. From the participants, I realized that I enjoy the administrator's role and taking on new challenges. I was amazed at the amount of change the two educational leaders, Connie and Kathy, were able to accomplish in a relatively short period of time. In an environment that was not conducive to change, they broke the barriers and made change happen.

I also detected a struggle between work and family issues reflected in Kathy and Christine. During our first interview, Kathy made no mention of the fact she was pregnant. However, the second interview revealed a very different side as she spoke often about her upcoming life change: expecting twins this summer. She pondered about how she would adjust to the new role. Christine also spoke often of her children. Handling multiple tasks such as proofreading and teaching made me question her career goals. She spoke about an independent project as a future goal. However, it appeared that her current work, while she put forth great effort, was more of a job and a way to earn extra income. I can relate to the situations as I attempted to balance work, family, and school responsibilities. I reflected on the reasons for taking on different projects and realized that although I learned a great deal from various roles, I was not in any set career path. It is exhausting balancing too many responsibilities and reporting to various people at multiple institutions. Their energy expressed in the interview helped me gain energy and inspiration. After reflecting upon women's roles in higher education, I decided that I would not sell out and take on yet another "job." I realized that I need to find a rewarding and challenging career in my field.

Fortunately I was able to find a position as an assistant professor of English and Communications at a small, private 4-year college. Typically I teach three or four courses per quarter, which include: Rhetoric and Public Issues, Research Writing, Business Communications, the

Teaching of Writing, Senior Seminar, Signature Course in Humanities, College Writing, and Speech. My experience pursuing a doctorate in educational leadership and organizational change awoke the leader within. Although all faculty members are responsible for serving on various committees, my thirst for constant learning and the desire to create change leads me in the direction of taking on many different leadership positions.

Since the university is small (approximately 1,200 students), the structure of the department includes both English and Communications. Since my interests lie in both areas, I have flexibility with course assignments and teach both English and Communications courses. A format I enjoy is the combination of teaching the College Writing (remedial writing) and Teaching of Writing courses. In this format, two courses meet jointly. The College Writing students are freshmen who scored low on the entrance exam and need remediation before matriculating into the regular curriculum. The Teaching of Writing students are juniors or seniors interested in pursuing a career in education. During the joint class I lecture to both groups in large- and small-group format with open discussions. A portion of the class is dedicated to peer review of writing of the College Writing students by the "teachers" of writing. This collaborative method is effective in the sense that the students have the opportunity to meet one-on-one with older students to discuss ways to improve writing. Another benefit of these one-on-one meetings is that the older students share experiences with the college, discuss challenges and benefits of the university, and discuss career goals. Comments from the students in the fall 2003 class revealed that both students enjoyed the format and grew in their understanding of the process [of] writing from working in collaboration.

Typically I also teach the Senior Seminar course three times per year. This is a required course for all students pursuing a bachelor's degree. Topics for the course change every year and have included Technology and Society and Postmodern Thought: Discussion and Discourse. The Senior Seminar is a course I enjoy teaching the most because of the flexibility in the design of the course. Since the majority of the students are seniors, there is a greater sense of commitment to discussion and completing of assignment. The dialogue is also engaging as students are encouraged to participate in dialogue and discussion. Following the theory of constructivist learning, it is explained that all members of the learning community should take an active role in their learning.

The courses I teach are reflective of my past experiences and current interests. Technology has always played a major role in my personal and professional career, and it is rewarding to see students "create" and present their vision in an oral presentation. For example, when assigning presentations that require visual aids, it is not a question of what can you do with technology, it is what you would like to do with technology in your presentation. Students have used multimedia such as incorporating MP3 music files, video clips, and Flash movies into their presentations. Similar to my belief in the value of technology, the power to create a product to share with others as a testimony of your ability and thoughts can be represented through technology.

Overall, my current position draws upon many of my past experiences. I have the ability to research, write, and present scholarly work; assist others in the learning process; and prepare others for a rewarding career. When teaching others course content materials, personal experiences related to my past work are often shared with the students. The learning process is dynamic, and as such I continue to grow as my students do. Presentations given to groups of students in my early role as student health educator in my undergraduate years began my preparation for teaching at the college level. Overall, every experience, both personal and professional, has helped me grow into the person and instructor I am today.

I also serve as the University Assessment Director and Student Internship Coordinator. Both positions allow me to assist in making university change in curriculum. The internship position plays into my desire to help students achieve their dream: obtaining a challenging position in the field of choice. Students are able to gain real-world experience in the professional world while still in college. It is very rewarding to know that I assisted students with their journey in pursuing a career. Additional projects I have worked on the past year include designing an education program, designing an English certificate program, assisting in the creation of an English website, and hiring and training new faculty members.

The road continues to wind as I reflect about the next transition in my life. Although I thoroughly enjoy teaching, I see myself taking on more of an administrative role in the future. I continue to research and write and have been fortunate to present several papers at national conferences. Reflecting back on Seurat's work, I now realize that every event, every experience shapes us into the people we are today. Continuing to grow and stretch in many areas allows me to continue my journey . . . oftentimes without a road map. However, I always seem to stop at rewarding areas along the way and continue the journey once more. A French painter who was a leader in the neo-Impressionist movement of the late 19th century, Georges Seurat is the ultimate example of the artist as scientist. Like Seurat, the qualitative researcher is an artist and a social scientist. Instead of dots or strokes of contrasting color on a canvas, the many experiences in my life, like Seurat's contrasting color, were used to create subtle changes in the formation of my life and career.

∽

In this example, we have a section of a story of an individual's lived experience through the words of the individual and co-constructed with the oral historian. This adds to the record on women's lives so often missing in traditional oral history approaches and so often forgotten. As with the example in Part I of this book, Leona's oral history, including women's voices augments the existing historical record. There are various ways to deconstruct the layers of the oral history in process. Consider the following case. Here the oral historian describes the context, summarizes the content of one interview, and then reflects on it. When beginning analysis and interpretation of Lynn's story, one might start with a theoretical frame with which to make sense of it. Feminist oral history would be a likely framework. As any good historian might do, look for themes, recurring issues, and points of conflict, or what does not seem to make sense, to begin analysis and interpretation. For a recent class exercise, members read Lynn's story and worked in small groups, then as a whole, to come up with a set of nine original themes and categories and then discussed as a whole the first round of categories, collapsing them into two: (1) Lynn's ability to grow and change and (2) Lynn's ability to be resilient despite personal change. Each group went on to write up their interpretations of these two themes as findings. This is one small example of oral history in action. Now let us turn to another example. In this next case a researcher reflects on the relationship with a participant, as well as the content of the remarks made in an interview.

CASE II.5.
∽

A Narrative Reflection on an Oral History Project

Alex M. Baryshnikov's Thoughts upon Interviewing Cora D. Humphrey:
First Interview

Almost instantly I knew whom I would interview for this assignment. I had read about her in *The New York Times* a few years before coming to Florida, while I was living in New York City. She had gained legendary status for teaching at the age of 86. The picture in my mind was a decrepit old woman directing lessons from a rocking chair. I wanted to see if such was the case. My primary concern, however, was to learn her thoughts on segregation and integration, particularly since she had lived as an educator in both dynamic worlds.

I learned from Miss Humphrey that she worked at Eland High School. I found the telephone number and called the school. A professional voice answered the phone, and when I asked for Miss Humphrey, the voice told me to hold on. The phone went silent for a few seconds. I choked on my saliva when I heard the next voice say, "Miss Humphrey." I was not expecting her to answer the phone! School was in session. I thought she would be in the middle of instruction directing students with her cane. I told her as much (okay, not all of what I thought!). She confirmed she was in class, but informed me that the principal had set up the private line in her room to accommodate her needs. I said a few insane things, which I do not recall because I was too excited, before making my request to visit. She explained she taught three 90-minute English honors classes beginning at 7:15 A.M. and said I was more than welcome to visit any of them, and afterwards, we could meet to discuss my needs. She repeatedly called me "darhlin'" ("darling" with a heavy Southern feminine drawl). We set a date, March 21st, a day I will never forget.

Monday morning I set out to meet the great Miss Humphrey. It was early. So early I felt like the birds were not up yet. I was barely awake, but moving, nonetheless. I sang without the radio for most of the 30-minute drive. Oddly, I began to get nervous. It was not that I was not prepared. I was. Yet, I wondered how truthful she would be given that she was a Southern elderly White woman and I, a younger, 6'5", educated Black man. I considered these as possible interview limitations, in addition to several others, including the notion that people interviewed may not be able to say what they think or may not be able to state their opinion in a clear way; respondents may be unwilling to discuss what they know; and that interviewing requires high-level questioning skills and an active interpretation. I also considered that time and distance could have mediated her memory. Only a few miles away, I felt so close to knowing and was unsure if I would get any information. I said a prayer and hoped for the best. As I pulled into the Eland High School parking lot, I looked for the main entrance. I found it, parked close by, got out of my car, and walked toward the door. I pulled it open and was greeted by a "darhlin'" lady who told me it was spring break and Miss Humphrey had left a note for me.

I stupidly forgot that we are on spring break—I apologize profusely. You are welcome to call me again, if you are not too angry with me. I may blow my brains out over my stupidity.

Miss Humphrey

Monday, March 27, 2006, we finally met. She walked over, no cane in sight, and shook my hand with a noticeably firm handshake. She appeared remarkably enthusiastic. If I were to guess by looking I would say she was in her 70s, nowhere near the 89 years she claims, despite the noticeable hump in her back. She's a small woman, about 5'1" tall and weighs approximately 100 pounds. Class had begun, and her students were seated.

As she walked around the room simultaneously taking attendance and checking homework journals, I observed the room. It was filled mostly with mementoes from the life of Miss Humphrey, thus rich in a way that only time as a teacher for 65-plus years would allow. The classroom had a homey feel to it, including scented candles, flowers, and a large throw rug. There were no signs of students' work displayed anywhere in the room, but lots of books on bookshelves along nearly every wall in the room. The books made the room seem class-like and a place of intellect. There were six tables, three on each side of the room, angled along the walls and one extending across the rear of the room.

There were four to five chairs at each table. A podium stood at the front and in the center of the room. A chair, that looked like it was from part of a dinette set, sat next to the podium. (This is the only image that I got almost right with my preconceptions, although the chair was not a rocker.)

"Pilgrim Sharing" was written on the board. Students had been asked to relate the human conditions revealed by the characters in the prologue to Chaucer's *Canterbury Tales* to their lives today. Each presented from the podium. Miss Humphrey sat in the chair next to the podium. I pulled up a fold-out chair and sat next to her. The lesson was remarkable and inspiring. So was our telling interview. Below is an excerpt.

Monday, March 27, 2006 Time: 12:30 P.M.

HUMPHREY: Alex, we never integrated the schools, we simply let Black children come to a White high school; it wasn't a question of integration. We just said, okay, "You Black children close down your Black school and you can come over here and go to a White school." You will lose your alma mater, you will lose your football team, you will lose your school's history, you will lose your individuality as a graduate of a good Black high school—you-are-bringing-nothing. You will take our alma mater, you will take our cheers, you will take our study course—not one that has come together, but you can now do ours—and if you don't understand that, you don't understand what part of the problem was. Oh yeah. Our English department went out to the Black high school here—this was in the '70s wasn't it, sweetheart? (*referring to the 30-year librarian, who interrupts*)

[Brief intermission]

I started to tell you our English department went out and met with the English department at Roe, which was the Black high school. There was an older teacher there, we had excellent meetings exchanging ideas, there was an older teacher there who walked with me—I bet you've never thought about this, either—out to the car one day and she said, "Black children grow up knowing about White stuff. They watch White television, they read White newspapers, they see White movies; they see a world run pretty much by Whites." She said, "You all don't know anything about us." I, I'd never been in a Black home. I was 30 years old; I'd never been in a Black home.

She said, "You don't know anything about us." That was gospel, my dear. We didn't. We took a bunch of children we knew nothing about [inaudible] but their, who they were, what their backgrounds were, their personal stuff, their home life. And we tried so hard, we were so dumb, we just tried so hard. A darling bright Black girl in the back of the room raised her hand one day and said, "Miss, it's okay if you say Black. I know I'm Black." Well, I wouldn't say Black to a child in a million years, it might hurt their feelings. We never wrote anything on the board that could be interpreted in the least way as offensive to a Black child. I tease mine now, saying we didn't even say "blackboard." We were really, really careful. We should have had a course then in standard spoken English. It would have done those children a world of good. They needed that in the job market. But we didn't want to imply there was anything they ever needed to learn; we never even thought about it. Out of a good heart we did a bunch of dumb stuff that made it harder, I think. But my children today, we talk about racial issues. They still say that they have teachers that they feel have racist attitudes toward Blacks and, um, the Caribbean culture, also. But my White children don't see that. And we talk about that from both points of view, but my Black children would say they see prejudice in this high school and my White children say no.

ALEX: How is it that you can talk among White people about racism with no Blacks present? I mean is that possible that you can have the conversation?

HUMPHREY: In my third period I don't have no Blacks. That class you visited I don't have a Black child in that class. So we can talk about White issues and Black issues and—

ALEX: And they do think racism exists.

HUMPHREY: My Black students do.

ALEX: What about the White students?

HUMPHREY: No, rarely do they say they see any evidence of it. And I say to my few Black children with teachers sometimes—but I remember one time in class one Black guy had done something really remarkably impressive, I'd read it in the paper, and I shared it with the children—this was a long time later, and I said, "This fine, young Black man," and one of my girls, a Black girl, said, "You know that's racist, you didn't have to identify him as a Black man." And I thought really that was sort of the point of the story, that he'd overcome some things that had been obstacles, but she felt that had been a racist remark. And I do think a lot of the young Blacks have a chip on their shoulder. You do, too.

ALEX: Hmmm. . . . (*pondering*).

HUMPHREY: I don't mean you have it, you understand that, too.

INTERVIEW SUMMARY BY ALEX

During our interview we were interrupted three times at length, with people dropping by to say hello. After the third interruption, I made the decision to conclude our interview. She thanked me. In the interview, on a very deep and personal level, we discussed preintegration and segregationist teaching practices. Because of her unique experience as a teacher for 65-plus years in the racially separate and racially inclusive worlds of education, she was my hope for knowing much of this information. She provided good information. The fact that she is still teaching makes the knowledge current. We also discussed her mother and father, her extended family, and her relation, connection, and understanding of Black people; her racist past, what keeps her going at 89, and her pleasures. She is highly critical of Black people. Notwithstanding her admitted inability to teach Black students, then and now, she seems to solely blame their social issues on "the chip on their shoulders."

THEMES AND REFLECTIONS FROM THIS FIRST INTERVIEW

After repeatedly listening to the tapes and constantly reading and rereading the interview transcripts, the idea is that, as the researcher becomes familiar with the data, slowly but surely categories "emerge" or become apparent. The data are reviewed, and the evaluator begins to see that the respondent has been talking about theme A, theme B, and so on. Pondering on these themes, the researcher finally comes to understand (interpret) that the respondent is talking about X. In this way of looking at analytical categories, the categories are "grounded" in the data. Standout themes grounded in the data from this interview are Miss H.'s commitment to children, her focus on living in the absence of family and in the old age of life, and her ill perception and understanding of Blacks, which is deeply entrenched in her past and to me arguably exemplifies racist behavior.

It is clear Miss Humphrey loves children. There is an unmistakable sincerity in her voice when she calls them endearing terms, like "darhlin'" or "sweetheart"; she cares about what they know, how they behave, and how they think. I learned these things after watching her teach for 90 minutes and also from our interview, when she said, "This morning I don't know if you were here when I mentioned this or not, but if you were, tell me so, but my first couple of kids who did the Knight and the Squire were very bored and negative with it and just kind of threw it away, and I had one of my fits about that, and I say, 'If you are bored with it, how does the audience feel?' They said, 'They are bored, too.' I said, 'That's right.' I said, 'Suppose you don't feel like making it energetic? What do you do? Well, you fake it!' I do professional speaking, I'm a motivational speaker besides. 'I'd like to say I'm bored with this myself, but you need to have that energy.' The next little girl that got up was top of the world, she just did it twice as good. Well, that just makes me laugh my pants off, that's so adorable. And kids do stuff like that all the time; nutty and very precious to me." The children, as she calls them, comfort what I perceive to be her loneliness. She's an only child; both of her parents are deceased, and she chooses not to maintain contact with any other family member. The children are her family. Her relationship with them is decidedly give and take. "I ask these kids, when I first get them, 'I will change your lives; how many of you believe, how many of you think you will change mine?' Not a one of them raise their hand. I said, 'Every day. Every day being with you changes my life.'" She says the children help her grow, they keep her grounded, but I discovered they also give her reason to live.

Miss Humphrey's life's focus has been her work. She calls herself a miracle and in our interview said, "I ought to be in a nursing home. I ought to be in assisted living. I ought to be having somebody look after me, and the fact that I am still able to drive my car to work every day 180 days out of the year is a miracle." She contends that working every day with students keeps her blood rushing, which allows her to stay healthy. When she's not busy working, she travels. "I've been everywhere—not Russia, not Alaska–every place else, and I like to go by myself." But whether she travels alone or with a companion, simply being on the go is what matters. She believes the opposite of an active life is one she's not ready to face, so work and travel keep her active and alive. Together they provide her focus for living.

Her active life, both past and present, has formed her sense of knowing. This takes me to a third theme that stood out in the interview: race relations. Although she was kind enough to agree to this interview and to discuss the topic of my choice, I sensed she was grateful for the interruptions. I also sometimes felt patronized by some of her comments. She said racism doesn't exist anymore, and her tone, during parts of our conversation, seemed to question my purpose for resurrecting what her words suggested she believes is a dead or nonissue. She seemed to imply that I was smarter than that. I also sensed the conversation dredged up memories she'd rather forget, including the death of her mother and father and her own racist past and behaviors. While I believe she is unduly critical of Black people, I also believe she believes Black students are smart. She thinks they make bad choices. She never considers the lessons she and others failed to teach as a possible reason for the bad decision making.

She admitted she and others didn't know how to academically engage Black students. "We never wrote anything on the board that could be interpreted in the least way as offensive to a Black child. I tease mine now, saying we didn't even say 'blackboard.' We were really, really careful. We should have had a course then in standard spoken English. It would have done those children a world of good. They needed that in the job market. But we didn't want to imply there was anything they ever needed to learn; we never even thought about it." The period in which she spoke was shortly after integration, but even today she still has a difficult time teaching Black students. Today, when she corrects Black students, she said, "I do it with humor."

I believed her when she said in our interview that, "Out of a good heart we did a bunch of dumb stuff that made it harder, I think." I also believe her cultural understanding, which is traditionally based, drove her practice. Times changed. She changed. Despite knowing that Black students had not been properly taught under her watch, she expected Black people to change. Today, she laments the plight of Black people and said, by way of explanation for their plight, "Blacks have a chip on their shoulder," "Blacks see themselves as disadvantaged," and "Half of them think they're going to be football or basketball players, a pathetic mentality." She used the words of a Black writer to bolster her claim,

"But that guy who, I don't know who the one it is, but who writes for the paper, he's very perceptive about the Blacks not, what's the word I want, not using the great abilities to promote themselves to accept doing drugs, dropping out of school, and getting girls pregnant. He says they accept that. They can't blame that on the White people! That's their own. He preaches that a lot better than I can tell you. And I am strong for that. But the Black children will say they are discriminated against in going to the office, being sent for referral, and things like that, and the White children will say that's not true, that's not true. I would probably say it's not true." Miss Humphrey represents what is, what was, and the complication of those things. I appreciated that she answered my questions. I refused to debate her answers; that was not my purpose for being here. However, I was saddened by some of them.

In this example we find an alternative type of narrative, which integrates selected sections of the interview into the narrative and includes the voice of the researcher/interviewer. To get to Miss Humphrey's story, Alex knew he would return for quite possibly several interviews. The issue of race came up serendipitously yet turned out to be a critical part of the final narrative and of the researcher's reflection on race and gender in oral history interviews. Alex's journal of thoughts became a foundation for thinking about social justice issues in the course of the project. In addition to interviews and writing oral history, journal writing is a helpful tool and an effective habit for the oral historian. Consider the technique of journal writing to augment the oral history in process.

JOURNAL WRITING FOR THE ORAL HISTORIAN AND FOR THE NARRATOR

A journal may be used as a qualitative research technique in qualitative studies and oral history projects by the interviewer and by the participant/narrator. For qualitative researchers, the act of journal writing may be incorporated into the research process to provide a dataset of the researcher's reflections on the research act, as well as the participant/narrator's reflections on the story being told. Participants in qualitative studies may also use journals to refine ideas, beliefs, and their own responses to the research in progress. Finally, journal writing between participants and researcher may offer the qualitative researcher yet another opportunity for triangulation of datasets at multiple levels. Journal writing has a long and reliable history in the arts and humanities, and qualitative researchers may learn a great deal from this. It is not by accident that artists, writers, musicians, dancers, therapists, physicians, poets, architects, saints, chefs, scientists, and educators use journal writing in their lives. Virtually in every field, one can find exemplars who have kept detailed and lengthy journals regarding their everyday lives and their beliefs, hopes, and dreams. I see journal writing as a powerful heuristic tool and research technique, and I discuss reasons for using a journal within qualitative research projects in order to do the following:

1. Refine the understanding of the role of the researcher through reflection and writing, much like an artist/choreographer might do.

2. Refine the understanding of the responses of participants in the study, much like a physician or health care worker might do.

3. Use a journal as an interactive tool of communication between the researcher and participants in the study, as a type of interdisciplinary triangulation of data.

4. View journal writing as a type of connoisseurship by which individuals become aware of their own thinking and reflection patterns and, indeed, as interviewers.

5. Elaborate on social justice issues concerning race, class, and gender through writing and reflection.

The notion of a comprehensive reflective journal in which the researcher addresses him- or herself is critical in qualitative work due to the fact that the researcher is the research instrument. Journal writing, although an ancient technique, is only now being used and talked about in the literature as a serious component in qualitative research projects. I have always seen journal writing as a major source of data. It is a dataset that contains the researcher's reflection on the role of the researcher, for example. It is a great vehicle for coming to terms with exactly what one is doing as a qualitative researcher. Often, qualitative researchers and oral historians are criticized for not being precise about what they do. I offer journal writing as one technique by which to accomplish the description and explanation of the researcher's role in the project. In addition, participants in an oral history often find a journal helpful for remembering experiences that connect to their present story. In every oral history project I am involved with as researcher/interviewer, I give a notebook to all participants to jot down things they recall postinterview.

Qualitative researchers and historians may also use reflective journals to write about problems that come up on a regular basis. Examples of problems include representations of interviews and field notes, co-construction of meaning with participants in the project who also keep journals, and issues related to the interpretation of each other's data. Sometimes deciding what goes into the narrative and what to leave out is a difficult matter. By reflecting on these issues and writing a journal of one's thoughts, one may more easily write a rationale for what is left in and what is left out. Often, we as oral historians and researchers are positioned outside the very people and situations we write about. Journal writing personalizes representation in a way that forces the researcher to confront issues of how a story from a person's life becomes a public text, which in turn tells a story. In other words, how do the researcher and the participant or participants in the project move from a blank page to sentence after sentence of description of a given set of experiences and responses and tell a story, the spine of qualitative work? Furthermore, how are we to make sense of this writing and understand how lived experience is represented by the writer/researcher and the participants? Many journal writers have weighed in on this question across disciplines.

Therapists view the journal as an attempt to bring order to one's experience and a sense of coherence to one's life. Behaviorists, cognitivists, and Jungian analysts have used journals in the process of therapy. The journal is seen as a natural outgrowth of the clinical situation in which the client speaks to the self. Most recently, Ira Progoff (1992) has written about keeping an intensive journal. Progoff developed a set of techniques that provide a structure for keeping a journal and a springboard for development. As a therapist himself, he has conducted workshops and trained a network of individuals to do workshops on keeping intensive journals to unlock one's creativity and come to terms with oneself. The intensive-journal method is a reflective, in-depth process of writing, speaking what is written, and, in some cases, sharing what is written with others. Feedback is an operative principle of the Progoff method. The individual needs to draw on inner resources to arrive at the understanding of the whole person; the journal is a tool to reopen the possibilities of learning and living. Progoff advocates:

1. Regular entries in the journal in the form of dialogue with oneself.

2. Maintaining the journal as an intensive psychological workbook in order to record all encounters of one's existence.

3. Some type of sharing of this growth through journal writing with others.

The method makes use of a special bound notebook divided into definite categories that include dreams, stepping-stones, and dialogues with persons, events, work, and the body. The writer is asked to reflect, free associate, meditate, and imagine that which relates to immediate experience. The latest version of his text (Progoff, 1992) is a testimonial to a solid example of techniques for keeping a journal. Obviously, anyone can write a journal without this structure. The value of the structure is that it forces reflection and recollection.

In fact, journal writing is so prevalent now that one only has to surf the Internet to see thousands of journal resources, examples, and personal histories online. For example, an online course on journal writing is offered by *www.higherawareness.com/journal-writing*; there are also a website entirely devoted to Ira Progoff's intensive journal workshop, chat rooms on journal writing, exemplars of diaries and journal writing, and literally thousands of resources. The reader of this book will be somewhat overwhelmed by the multitude of sources. As with anything on the Internet, you will have to sift through to see what is best for your learning style. In general, the common thread that unites all these resources on the Internet is the agreement that journal writing is a way of getting in touch with yourself in terms of reflection, catharsis, remembrance, creation, exploration, problem solving, problem posing, and personal growth. All of these are habits to develop in order to improve the act and the art of interviewing.

Although journal writing has its seeds in psychology, sociology, and history, I rely on social psychology and the symbolic interactionists to understand the use of the journal. Symbolic interactionists have historically argued that we all give meaning to the symbols we encounter in interacting with one another. Interpretive interactionists go a step further in that the act of interpretation is a communication act with one or more interactors. Basically, the art of journal writing and subsequent interpretations of journal writing produce meaning and understanding that are shaped by genre, the narrative form used, and personal cultural and paradigmatic conventions of the writer, who is the researcher, participant, and/or co-researcher. As Progoff (1992) notes, journal writing is ultimately a way of getting feedback from ourselves, and in so doing, it enables us to experience in a full and open-ended way the movement of our lives as a whole and the meaning that follows from reflecting on that movement.

Journal writing allows one to reflect, to dig deeper, if you will, into the heart of the words, beliefs, and behaviors we describe in our journals. The clarity needed for writing down our thoughts allows us to step into our inner minds and reach further into interpretations of the behaviors, beliefs, and words we write.

For example, a student conducting a mini-study in a qualitative methods class wrote in her journal and described some of her inner thoughts:

> I am a bit wary of this research. . . . Am I really a researcher because I am taking a class? Can I ever hope to portray what someone else believes or at least says she believes? How will I know if I am being fair? Will I be able to trust this person? Will she trust me? Why should she trust me? Am I being too critical of myself? I am waiting here, and she is already 20 minutes late. I hope she gets here soon. . . . Here she comes. Now I try to capture this person's thoughts on why she is an administrator. . . .

As we look at this journal entry, one can easily see the learner/ researcher in training, asking questions that cause reflection on various issues in the research process. She is beginning to know more about herself and her strengths and weaknesses. This alone can make a person more reflective and more appreciative of the process of telling someone else's story through oral history.

Here is another example from J. D., an experienced teacher of some 15 years who teaches middle school in a metropolitan area. What an amazing example of her thoughts on teaching:

I love these kids . . . most from broken homes, most thinking I am their parent, advisor, guardian, good cop, teacher, analyst, and coach. I am trying to get them to read more . . . comic books, novels, go to the library, and then get them to write about this. I think I will go for the two-page report idea again. It gives me something to reinforce their understanding of what they read and to give them some feedback. I am worried about P. He is always skipping class these days, and although I know his brother is home from prison, I wish he would come back to school. I will talk to the principal about this today if I don't forget. I also want to design a new way of evaluating my class without the letter grades we are stuck with. I am reading about the use of portfolios in classroom assessment, and I think I will try it this month and get the kids to plan it with me.

This is a good example of what journal writing can do to assist a person in the eventual construction of a narrative. In addition, H. H. let me see her journal entries. I am going to use only one of her examples regarding a problem in her classroom.

Once again I have to deal with M. Why is he refusing to write in class and why is he afraid to tell me what is bothering him? He has done this before but we could always talk this out before . . . I am taking a class right now that relates to this directly. . . . None of the books or papers is helping me so I am just going ahead and going to try a home visit to talk to his Mom and see if she can help. . . . Since I started visiting parents who were unable to come to teacher conferences, I am humbled by what I am learning. . . . M's mother is working three jobs to keep the family of three children and herself together. . . . I wonder if I would have her courage at this point? She has told me that M is getting in with the "wrong crowd" and has been involved in questionable activities, which is why he is skipping school so often. Even sending someone to check on this has not yielded any positive results. She said she thought this was due to more than "being a teenager" but felt that there were no strong role models for him at home. No relatives live nearby. I brought some of M's work to show her, and she felt a bit reassured that at least he was doing something, though she added that "he could do better." I decided I would talk to him tomorrow and ask him to help me organize the class project on voting in the November elections. I felt conflicted upon leaving the house, for I feared that M's Mom needed to talk to someone about her kids and that I wasn't very much of a help at all. I do feel more inspired to be better at letting the kids take over more of the responsibility for class projects. Actually it was M who taught me this month when he volunteered to lead the book circle discussion.

When I look at this entry I can see someone still alive and thinking about teaching in a way that makes the basic questions of what and how to teach take on a renewed meaning. Many journal writers agree that journal writing is an effective tool to spark reflection. In addition, journal writing can assist in the daily practice of writing, the heart and soul of the narrative written portrayal, the eventual goal of any oral history. Journals are a powerful dataset for the oral historian and any qualitative researcher. In addition, multiple and various documents serve to provide more information and texture in many oral history projects.

DOCUMENTS AS DATA

The use of selected documents to provide a rich texture for understanding someone's history is an age-old technique. The letters, notes, and written official documents used in many oral history projects provide a solid backdrop for checking the actual state of things. For example, in the 9/11 oral histories of New York City firefighters, the call sheets, the phone logs, and the lists of medications and on-site

emergency services provided have helped to make the reader realize the social context of what was occurring on the site at Ground
Zero and nearby. Recently, documents have come into prominence
as part of qualitative data analysis. Altheide, Coyle, DeVriese, and
Schneider (2008) have written extensively on emergent qualitative
document analysis (QDA), sometimes also called ethnographic content analysis. So as not to confuse the issue, here I discuss the QDA
as a technique that is most useful in augmenting the analysis and
interpretation of oral history. In the document analysis, it is helpful to focus on the content matter of the document and the interaction, if one exists, between the document and the participant in
the oral history project. QDA is thought of as an orientation toward
research. It helps to make the past vividly connected to the present
in many cases. Themes and relationships are also part of analyzing
documents that may augment our understanding of a person's life,
for example. In the example used earlier of Lynn's story, she provided many memos and documents she had created in previous and
current work. She selected them to provide examples from her years
in publishing and then from her most recent career shift into the
academic world. These documents were part of her portfolio of life,
so to speak. So documents for the oral historian are an extension of
the person. They merit exploration and searching for understanding.
The historian would use the same approach to documents as that
used to transcripts:

1. Find major themes.
2. Build categories of key concepts found in the documents.
3. Look for what is missing.

As qualitative researchers in general work toward building a model
of what occurred in the study, so do oral historians. Often data do not
speak for themselves. The researcher interprets those data to assist
the reader of the report in understanding what was discovered.

In the preceding sections, I have reviewed some major points
on interviewing, journal writing, and QDA for the oral historian as

a qualitative researcher. Interviewing, for the oral historian, can be seen as a creative act dependent on developing good habits of mind. As an oral historian in training, you might develop the good habit of **being prepared**:

1. **With technology.** Before going out into the field, check all your gear, test your gear, and be sure it is functioning to your satisfaction.

2. **In terms of content of the interview.** Know your questions inside and out. Know the content area you will be dealing with during the interview. For example, I recently began a study of female school superintendents. Before even locating and selecting participants for the study, I did a thorough literature search for the writings on this topic between the years 2000 and 2006. I checked government statistics and documents on the demographics of school superintendents and did a search of *Dissertation Abstracts International* to find the latest research on the topic. This enabled me to understand more fully the social context of female school superintendents. This also helped me to craft better questions for the oral history project as a whole.

3. **With some practice interviewing or a pilot study** to test out your questions.

4. **To encounter problems in the social world.**

   a. The interviewer shows up for the appointed interview, but an emergency has called away the participant. What do you do?

   b. The interview is in progress, and the tape recorder malfunctions. What do you do?

5. **To keep a journal of the project** and to encourage your participants to keep a journal.

6. **To read a great deal.** Read about everything that relates to the person you are interviewing. Understand her or him in the social context, the demographics of the person's life, and so forth. Also read about the art and craft of interviewing.

7. **To listen** to what is being said.

8. **For the unexpected.** By this I mean, because the social world is always active rather than static, being prepared for all those things that the chaos of the social world can bring. They may include, to name just a few, participants who change the interview date or the interview questions, weather conditions that may cancel the flight you need to get to the participant in the study, computer or equipment malfunctions, and your own health problems.

Goldberg (2005) stated that writing is 90% listening. If you as the interviewer are a good listener, you have the opportunity to hear the data by listening meaningfully and in depth. You may continue that listening as you write. One pitfall interviewers in training often remark on is the fact that, after they had completed the first interview, they noticed that they as interviewers talked a lot and interrupted the speaker. Thus a good habit to develop to ensure a quality interview is to stay silent, let the narrator speak, and allow the interview to proceed. It is perfectly fine to be still, be quiet, and let the story emerge. Listen to what is being said.

DOCUMENTS, ARTIFACTS, AND PHOTOGRAPHS TO AUGMENT ORAL HISTORY REPORTS

Although interviewing is the major technique of qualitative work in most cases, and although journal writing as a research technique works well for many to enrich a project, the importance of documents, artifacts, and photographs cannot be overstated. Documents enrich any study, especially while capturing some portion of history. To use the example of Hurricane Katrina once again, the well-known filmmaker Spike Lee constructed a documentary film about Katrina called *When the Levees Broke: A Requiem in Four Acts*, which aired on the Home Box Office network (HBO). Information on this film is also available at *www.hbo.com/docs/programs/whentheleveesbroke/interview.html*. Following is an interview with Spike Lee (n.d.) on the project. Lee reviewed many newscasts, documents, and artifacts and interviewed survivors of Katrina on the site immediately after it happened, and he stayed on to capture the various stories. The result was the 4-hour documentary. Here are some of his remarks on the project, which appear on the HBO website:

SPIKE LEE: When Hurricane Katrina went through New Orleans or around it, I was in Venice, Italy, at a film festival. . . . It was around that time that I decided that I would like to do this. And as soon as I got back to New York, I called up [HBO's] Sheila Nevins, and we met, and she agreed to go forward. What many people say in this film is that what happened in New Orleans is unprecedented. Never before in the history of the United States has the federal government turned its back on its own citizens in the manner that they did, with the slow response to people who needed help.

    Recently, there was another horrific earthquake, a national disaster in Indonesia. And, once again, the United States government was there within 2 days. Now it's great that we were in Indonesia in 2 days. But . . . let's get a globe (*laughs*), and see what the distance [is] between the United States and Indonesia, and to New Orleans, and the people in the whole Gulf region.

HBO: When you first set foot on the ground, was it what you expected? Were you prepared for what you saw?

SPIKE LEE: Anyone who has been to New Orleans will automatically tell you that what you saw on television, the pictures, they can't really describe the scale of the devastation. When you go to the Lower Ninth Ward, it looks—Hiroshima must have [looked] like that. Nagasaki. Beirut. Berlin after it was bombed in World War II. That's the way the Lower Ninth Ward looks like, and a lotta other places in New Orleans.

    People in New Orleans are up in arms about progress. People wanna move back. New Orleans was a predominantly African American city, and its Black citizens were dispersed to 46 other states. People wanna come home, but there's nowhere for them to live. They wanna work. The thing is just all messed up. I would not wanna be Mayor Ray Nagin. That has [to be] the next hardest job in this country besides the President of the United States, being the mayor of New Orleans.

HBO: Why do you think the response was what it was?

SPIKE LEE: Well, I would just say, what Kanye West expressed, that George Bush doesn't care about Black people. Many people think it had nothing to do with race, it had more to do with class. You have a large population who happened to be poor, and if they did vote they didn't vote Republican anyway. Everybody was on vacation. Ms. Rice was buying Ferragamo shoes on Madison Avenue while people were drowning, then went to see *Spamalot*. Cheney was on vacation. Bush was on vacation, and even when the President cut short his vacation, he did not fly directly to New Orleans. He did not fly directly to the Gulf region. He had the pilot of Air Force One do a flyover.

Politicians do many things that are symbolic. And people might say well, what's the good if it's just symbolic? Sometimes there's a lotta good in symbolism. In 1965 with Hurricane Betsy, then President Lyndon B. Johnson flew to New Orleans, and went to the Lower Ninth Ward. He shined a flashlight in his face in the dark and said, I'm Lyndon B. Johnson, I'm the President of the United States and we care about you. George Bush did not feel he had to do that. He showed up late, and the damage had been done already.

One of the things I hope this documentary does is remind Americans that New Orleans is not over with, it's not done. Americans responded in record numbers to help the people of the Gulf Coast, but let's be honest. Americans have very, very short attention spans. And, I'll admit there was eventually a thing called Katrina fatigue. But if you go to New Orleans, only one-fourth of the population is there. People are still not home. So hopefully, this documentary will bring this fiasco, this travesty, back to the attention of the American people. And maybe the public can get some politician's ass in the government to move quicker, and be more efficient in helping our fellow American citizens in the Gulf region.

HBO: Has this forever changed the way people think about New Orleans?

SPIKE LEE: I think when we look back on this many years from now, I'm confident that people are gonna see what happened in New

Orleans as a defining moment in American history. Whether that's pro or con is yet to be determined. And that's one of the reasons why I wanted to do this film.

I am using this example to indicate how oral histories may be told in various ways. In this case, a documentary was created by the director, Lee, who created the four acts from multiple sources, such as documents, artifacts, photographs, and personal stories.

Oral history may also benefit from the use of artifacts and documents, such as a person's journal left for future generations, wills, marriage certificates, and various photographs. In fact, many websites are in operation currently that encourage the use of photography for documenting one's life story or a portion of it. One well-known site that can be instructive is *www.photovoice.org*, for the organization Photovoice. This organization encourages the use of documentary photography by helping those left on the margins to document their lives. Currently Photovoice has projects in 12 countries, pioneering the use of photography with refugees, children, orphans, the homeless, and HIV/AIDS victims. Their locations include Macedonia, Russia, United Kingdom, Sri Lanka, Ethiopia, Cambodia, India, and Ecuador. Personnel consult with many nongovernment organizations (NGOs), such as foundations and UNICEF. The mission of Photovoice is a social justice mission to bring about positive social change. Members encourage photography and teach photography to individuals so as to enable them to document their lives and potentially generate income. Photovoice personnel are trying to sensitize the viewer to the plight of various outsiders, such as the homeless, for example. Because we are constantly viewing the visual image somewhere—on the Web, on television, in cinemas—we risk saturation and, worse, indifference. By purposefully using photography, we may more fully tell a story to those who will listen. There is a growing body of literature on the use of photography as a research technique. Often, photography is considered an archival strategy. We may find photographs and other documents in archives. Archives are a good resource for oral history.

Archival strategies are always valuable and useful for the qualitative researcher in general and the oral historian in particular. For example, a narrative can be greatly enriched with either public archival records or personal archival records. Public archives include libraries, tombstones, registries, hospital and police records, school records, commercial documents, and actuarial documents, to name a few. Private documents may include items and artifacts such as letters, notebooks, photographs within documents, and so forth. For a more detailed treatment of archival documents, see Lofland, Snow, Anderson, and Lofland (2006). We now have access to large amounts of information through the use of technology, so many archival documents are available for the asking.

SUMMARY

In this section of the book the major techniques of oral history were discussed. Examples were included to illustrate how these techniques may be used in narrative form. Oral history interviews, some with a suggestion of analytical interpretations, were included by the oral historian in question. Journal writing, documents, and photographs were also discussed as viable techniques relating to design and tension in oral history and other qualitative research projects.

PERFORMANCE EXERCISES

1. Write three pages in your journal in a dialogue format with yourself and write about what you wish to learn from the narrator in your oral history project.

2. Write three pages about your grandparents. If they are available to be interviewed, try an oral history interview with them.

3. Write three pages about your high school experience, which defined who you are today.

4. Photograph someone in your family and write about what you see in the photograph.

SELECTED READINGS

To improve your knowledge of interviewing skills and document and artifact collection, these books may be helpful.

Berg, B. L. (2007). *Qualitative research methods for the social sciences* (6th ed.). Boston: Pearson.

Cole, A. L., & Knowles, J. G. (2001). *Lives in context: The art of life history research.* New York: Alta Mira Press.

Janesick, V. J. (2004). *"Stretching" exercises for qualitative researchers* (2nd ed.). Thousand Oaks, CA: Sage.

Kvale, S., & Brinkmann, S. (2009). *InterViews: Learning the craft of qualitative research interviewing* (2nd ed.). Thousand Oaks, CA: Sage.

McCracken, G. (1988). *The long interview.* Newbury Park, CA: Sage.

Metzler, K. (1989). *Creative interviewing.* Englewood Cliffs, NJ: Prentice Hall.

Mishler, E. G. (1986). *Research interviewing: Context and narrative.* Cambridge, MA: Harvard University Press.

PART III

༄

BALANCE AND COMPOSITION

Becoming an Oral Historian

All history becomes subjective;
in other words, there is properly
no history; only biography.
—RALPH WALDO EMERSON

INTRODUCTION

Like the choreographer whose aim is to communicate a story of some kind to an audience, the oral historian also has to communicate a story. This means that writing is critical. Like the choreographer and the dancer, who train the body to perform, the prospective oral historian also is in training, particularly as a writer. In fact, writing is an athletic activity in the same way that dance and choreography are athletic activities. To write oral history, as in dance, you are engaging your mind, your memory, and your body parts, such as the hands, muscles, nervous system, spine, joints, eyes, ears, and brain. Even as I sit at my computer writing this book, I feel the strain on my eyes, the restlessness of my spine, the right hand and arm pinching, the legs anxious to get up and move. I notice the physical changes, which affect the mental changes, as I write, and so will you as you train to do oral history. I notice that I am thirsty while writing, so I stop and take a break. I notice hunger and the need for some protein. So will you as you begin this exciting journey.

A student asked me recently, How do I know I can even do oral history? Do I have the qualities needed, and can I identify what is needed for a good oral history? So I turned the questions back to him and asked him to tell me of his qualities that already have prepared him for doing oral history. This began a class dialogue on the qualities that may serve the oral historian and the characteristics of oral history. The following is what we agreed on as characteristics of oral history that can serve as guidelines to think about as you become an oral historian in the field:

- Oral history is holistic. Even if you are telling a vignette of someone's life, that vignette gives the entire picture of the person's life.

- Oral history, by virtue of telling a story, looks at relationships.

- Oral history usually depends on face-to-face immediate interactions.

- Oral history, like all qualitative work, demands time for analysis equal to the time spent in the field.

- Oral history acknowledges ethical issues that may arise in the interview.

- Oral history relies on the researcher as the research instrument.

- Oral history seeks to tell a story as it is, without reference to prediction, proof, control, or generalizability.

- Oral history incorporates a description of the role of the oral historian/researcher.

- Oral history incorporates informed consent and release forms or any formal documentation needed to protect persons involved in the oral history.

- Oral historians check back with participants in a member check to share transcripts and converse about the meaning of data.

- Oral historians develop trust and rapport with the narrators and respect the information given.

- Oral historians read widely and do all that is possible to understand the social context of the person being interviewed.

- Oral historians use all sorts of data. Even though oral history is a qualitative research technique, demographic information, documents, and other pertinent information may be used.

- Oral historians write every day and practice writing on a regular basis.

- Oral historians have deep appreciation for history.

- Oral historians may use the technology of the day, such as the Internet, and learn to tell a story from sources such as YouTube, blogs, written and posted diaries and journals, letters, and any other documentation.

- Oral historians may use photography and film to capture someone's lived experience.

- Oral historians may decide to tell the narrator's story using poetry or other art forms found in documents or in the transcripts or may craft their own poetry or use other art forms as well in the storytelling.

- Oral historians, by virtue of doing oral history research, are gaining knowledge and insight into the human condition by understanding some aspect of someone else's lived experience.

- Oral historians, by understanding one person's life in its complexity, come to understand more fully the context and community of which that person is a part.

This information, of course, is not new, but as individuals discover this for themselves, they can set about the task of becoming oral historians.

Continuing with the thread of what qualities the oral historian might develop, it seems that, like the qualitative researcher, an oral historian must be comfortable with ambiguity to begin with. When you write someone's story, you embark on a journey that will take many twists and turns. If I have learned anything in my work as a qualitative researcher and oral historian, it is that there is no uninteresting story! People have stories to tell, but very few have been asked to tell them. When asked, you may be surprised at what the story evolves into. I like to think of writing, oral history, choreography, and qualitative research as art forms. As such, the level of interpretation is up to the performer/writer and choreographer/oral historian. Stories can save lives by virtue of the telling of the story and through the artistry of the narrative. Continuing with our discussion of the possible qualities of the oral historian, we came up with the following:

- Oral historians should be comfortable with ambiguity.
- Oral historians should be above-average writers.
- Oral historians should be good listeners.
- Oral historians should be sensitive to ethical concerns in any study.
- Oral historians should get in sync with the interviewee/narrator's pace rather than rush things along.
- Oral historians should ask sensitive questions with care.
- Oral historians should not lead the witness.
- Oral historians should not interrupt the thoughts of the person being interviewed.
- Oral historians should expect the unexpected.
- Oral historians should write on a regular basis to sharpen narrative writing skills.
- Oral historians should practice using technology in all of its forms.
- Oral historians may have the opportunity to capture the stories of those left on the periphery of society and so contribute to various social justice projects and give voice to individuals who may have never been able to tell their stories previously.
- Oral historians acknowledge testimony as one kind of oral history.

As you can see, these are qualities common to qualitative researchers in general. For the oral historian, they take center stage, because we often are dealing with interviews that may have the potential to raise some social justice question, which in turn may make some readers of the oral history uncomfortable. One could easily say about oral history what the great North American labor leader Mother Jones said of her work: She noted it was her business "to afflict the comfortable and comfort the afflicted" (based on a quote from humorist Finley Peter Dunne). In fact, many oral histories do just that. See the recent 9/11 oral histories of New York City firefighters or the oral histories of Hurricane Katrina victims for recent stories of this nature. The World Wide Web has multiple sites of oral histories of 9/11 survivors and of Hurricane Katrina survivors, eyewitnesses, and first responders. Furthermore, looking at the oral history testimony of survivors of the Holocaust, one cannot help but be shaken. See the U.S. Holocaust Memorial Museum website (*www.ushmm.org*) for a collection called Life After the Holocaust to see oral history at its most profound. By the way, this site contains valuable archives, including an international database of oral history testimonies.

WRITING UP THE NARRATIVE

Many of my students tell me they want to write a novel, finish their dissertations in record time, or even become freelance writers. When I hear this, I ask, "How many hours per day are you writing? What is your writing schedule?" As you might imagine, many look at me astounded. But the writing process, like choreography and dance, takes practice. I also like to suggest that writing be done every day, preferably at the same time. For example, in my case, I am definitely a morning person, so I write as soon as possible in the morning and for as long as possible.

This is a way to establish a habit of mind, heart, and body. In dance, the dancer and choreographer work out every day to keep the habits of body and mind sharp. My meditation teacher always says it takes 30 days to develop a habit. So I ask you here to write every day for 30 days and see what you can do as an oral historian in training practicing narrative writing. Then take another 30 days to work just on the Web, becoming familiar with the sites that describe oral history, which have available tapes and videos, and actually take time needed to view and listen to completed projects.

But what can be said about style? Every writer has or needs to develop a style, and oral historians have as many styles as one can imagine. In the past, oral history was thought to be completed by doing some interviews on tape and storing them in a library or an archive open to a few users. Today this practice has become nearly obsolete because of the explosion of media and the availability of computers, cell phones that record photos and video for up to 1 hour, and other multimedia materials. In fact, the digital evolution/revolution will soon make other modes obsolete. Also, today we need to face the fact that we have little privacy. Someone walking by with a video camera could be taking your picture even if aiming for some tourist site. Such photos may end up having remarkable repercussions and consequences. For example, we would not have known about the Rodney King case in Los Angeles were it not for a tourist with a video camera. The repercussions of that case included the initiation of long-term scrutiny of the Los Angeles Police Department. So we have the capability to document life histories or portions of those histories presently in a way that was impossible even 20 years ago. My point is that when you write your final narrative of the oral history project, you may be assisted by the technology of the day, as well as by other forms of representation.

Writing up the narrative story depends on the interview transcripts, any documents being analyzed, and any other supporting datasets such as photographs and the researcher's reflective journal, as well as any observations on the scene. Documents may be provided by the narrator of the oral history or discovered by the oral historian. These may help to fill out the context of the story. Likewise, the researcher's reflexive journal is a valuable tool. I have written earlier (Janesick, 1999, 2004) on the importance of the researcher's reflexive journal. Let us turn once again to that topic. In the previous section of this book, we looked at two sample journal entries. The importance of the researcher's reflexive journal is further discussed in relation to its strength in developing the habit of reflexivity.

THE RESEARCHER'S REFLEXIVE JOURNAL

Journal writing as a reflexive research activity has been called *reflexive journaling* by many sociologists and researchers in training. It has been most used by qualitative researchers in the social sciences and other fields, as these professionals are seeking to describe a given social setting or a person's life history in its entirety. Qualitative research has a long history of its own that includes discussion of the techniques of the qualitative researcher. Reflexive journaling has been one of the regularly described and often used techniques (Janesick, 2004). It has proven to be an effective tool for understanding the processes of qualitative research more fully, as well as the experiences, mind-sets, biases, and emotional states of the researcher. Thus it may serve to augment any oral history reporting. This inclusion of the description of the role of the researcher and any reflections on the processes of the oral history project can be a valuable dataset.

Many qualitative researchers advocate the use of a reflexive journal at various points in the research project time line. To begin with, a journal is a remarkable tool for any researcher to use to reflect on the methods of a given work in progress, including how and when certain techniques are used in the study. Likewise, it is a good idea to track the thinking processes of the researcher and the participants in a study. In fact, writing a reflexive journal on the role of the researcher in any given qualitative project is an effective means to describe and explain research thought processes. Often qualitative researchers are criticized **for not explaining exactly how they conducted a study**. The reflexive journal writing of a researcher is one device that assists in developing a record of how a study was designed, why certain techniques were selected, and subsequent ethical issues that evolved in the study. A researcher may track in a journal the daily workings of the study. For example, did the participant change an interview appointment? How did this subsequently affect the flow of the study? Did a serious ethical issue emerge from the conduct of the study? If so, how was this described, explained, and resolved? These and other such questions are a few examples of the types of prompts for the writer. In addition, this emphasizes the importance of keeping a reflexive journal throughout the entire project (in this case, an oral history project).

If the reader checks recent dissertations completed and catalogued in *Dissertation Abstracts International*, it is easy to see that many recent dissertations include the use of a reflexive journal. The inclusion of the use of the reflexive journal as part of the data collection procedure indicates to some extent the credibility and trustworthiness of this technique. Does it not also act as a source of credibility and descriptive substance for the overall project? As a research technique, the reflexive journal is user friendly and often instills a sense of confidence in beginning researchers and a sense of accomplishment in experienced researchers. Many researchers verify that the use of a reflexive journal makes the acts of interviewing, observing, and taking field notes much more fluid. Researchers who use the reflexive journal often become more reflective actors and better writers. Writing in a journal every day instills a habit of mind that can only help in the writing of the final research report.

In beginning the researcher's reflexive journal, regardless of the project, it is always useful to supply all the basic descriptive data in each entry. Information such as the date, time, place, participants, and any other descriptive data should be registered in order to provide accuracy in reporting later in the study. Especially in long-term projects, the specific evidence that locates members and activities of the project can become most useful in the final analysis and interpretation of the research findings. Now let us turn to the history of the reflexive journal, and the creation of a reflexive journal, which are also critical aspects of the journaling process.

Journal writing began from a need to tell a story. Famous journal writers throughout history have provided us with eminent examples and various categories of journals (see Progoff, 1992). Journals can be written from the perspective of chronicler, traveler, creator, apologist, confessor, or prisoner, as Mallon (1995) describes. No matter what orientation is taken by the reflexive journal writer, it is generally agreed that reflexive journal writing is utilized to provide clarity, to organize one's thoughts and feelings, and to achieve understanding. Thus the oral history researcher has a valuable tool in reflexive journal writing.

Journal writing has its seeds in psychology, sociology, and history, and one can rely on social psychology and the symbolic interactionists for an understanding of the use of the journal. In addition, what Denzin (2001) calls "interpretive interactionism" is a useful tool for understanding the reflexive journal. Symbolic interactionists have historically argued that we all give meaning to the symbols we encounter in interacting with one another. Interpretive interactionists go a step further in that the act of interpretation is a communication act with one or more interactors. In journal writing, one is in a sense interacting with oneself.

Basically, the art of journal writing and subsequent interpretations of journal writing produce meaning and understanding, which are shaped by genre, the narrative form used, and the personal, cultural, and paradigmatic conventions of the writer who is the researcher, participant, and/or co-researcher. As Progoff (1992) notes, journal writing is ultimately a way of getting feedback from ourselves. In so doing, this enables us to experience in a full and open-ended way the movement of our lives as a whole and the meaning that follows from reflecting on that movement.

We might ask why we should invest the time in journal writing. Journal writing allows us to reflect, to dig deeper into the heart of the words, beliefs, and behaviors we describe in our journals. The act of writing down our thoughts will allow us to step into our inner minds and to reach further for clarity and interpretations of the behaviors, beliefs, and words we write. Journal writing also allows the training of a writer as a researcher in progress who is writing about a research project in progress. The journal becomes a tool for training the research instrument, the person. Because qualitative social science relies heavily on the researcher as research instrument, journal writing can only assist researchers in reaching their goals in any given project. Let us turn now to an example of a reflective journal entry from Jody J. Jamison, a doctoral student returning to do research. (This was a class assignment.)

CASE III.1.
ᙡ
A Researcher's Reflective Journaling on Her Autobiography and What Brought Her to Do Research
BY JODY J. JAMISON

As I think about my life, the one image that continues to recur is the action character, Optimus Prime—the protagonist of the autobots in the cartoon *Transformers*. The Transformers are a robotic society whose planet is destroyed, and survivors, in searching for a place to live, find Earth. According to Optimus Prime, the people of Earth have the capacity for great compassion and great discovery. To meld into earthly society, Optimus and his autobots take on many forms, such as automobiles, trucks, and helicopters. This enables them to move swiftly through our world in a form to which humans are accustomed in order to avoid frightening them. Unfortunately, along with the autobots, led by Optimus Prime, come the decepticons and their leader Megatron. Megatron comes to Earth, not to become part of human society but to replace it with a society plagued by oppression and despotism in which he would be leader. As [the name of] Megatron's team (the decepticons) would imply, they deceive in order to destroy, and their purpose for transforming into familiar forms is not to avoid frightening humans but, rather, to deceive them. Of course, Optimus is always searching for ways to oppose Megatron. Since Megatron matches Optimus in strength and leadership, there is an unwritten understanding between the two giants that good and evil will always coexist. Therefore, it is the goal of Optimus to present pressure at every step in order to mitigate the effects of Megatron's oppressive leadership. Thus the Transformers under Optimus's leadership keep vigilant watch over those who cannot resist the powers of Megatron and his decepticons as they await his call to action: Autobots: Roll out!

Like Optimus Prime, my life has transformed from wife and mother to teacher, from teacher to advocate, and, more recently, from advocate to critical theorist. Also like Optimus Prime, I have transformed into a vehicle for change and, in the process, have become part of a convoy to change the system.

IN THE BEGINNING . . .

I was born at the end of the Baby Boomer generation in 1964 as the youngest of three children born to a traditional middle-class family. I say "traditional" because the image of the average family of the 1950s consisted of a mother and father, 2.5 children, and a dog that all lived in a house surrounded by a white picket fence. As the ".5" member of the family, I was reminded frequently that children are to be seen and not heard. My older siblings always seemed to have more privileges, more freedom, and less responsibility. Household chores always seemed to be relegated to the person at the end of the line, and when disaster struck, it was always I who had caused it. But I suppose being the youngest had its advantages, too. Relatives continued to dote on me, pinch my cheeks, and bask in the misconception that I knew little of what was going on in the world. Therefore, I was able to "play dumb" whenever I became bored with the conversation and able to exit without anyone being offended. I learned early in life that it is wise to maintain the image you want people to have of you until you are ready to reveal a different image.

While I was born into a traditional family, my life was anything but traditional. When I was very young, my father began traveling a great deal when his company appointed him to train foreign workers to operate oil refineries in their native countries. Because he always put his family before business, he made sure that we went where he went. As a result, my young life is filled with stories and memories from countries ranging from south of the border to the Middle East. Though many images from my childhood come to mind, the one I remember with the most pride involves a group of orphans. This instance, I believe, is what set a course for the rest of my life.

TRANSFORMATION FROM CHILD TO AWARE CITIZEN

In 1968, life in Latin America was, at times, treacherous. Political regimes changed hands overnight as bloody, guerrilla-like battles spilled over into the streets, where innocent children often fell dead as stray bullets missed their adult targets. As I heard popping noises throughout the night, I asked my mother what I was hearing. She always reassured me I was safe by telling me that "It's just firecrackers exploding. The Spanish are such festive people." While I wanted to believe her, I didn't. I could see the despair in the children's faces; I could smell the gunpowder every morning; I noticed when people were suddenly missing from the town. These often senseless revolutions impoverished an already impoverished people and left children without parents, without food, and without hope. As a result, children had the task of gathering food and fending for themselves. Because they were small, they could steal food from vendors and be gone very quickly, thus narrowly escaping the fatal outcome of their parents. Even as a young child, I understood that I was privileged and, on some unknown level, I felt guilty about that. As the streets became more dangerous, children learned to stay hidden by day and active by night. It was on one of those nights that I made my first transformation.

My father left a weekly food allowance for our cook—and my personal friend—Alba. She prepared the most delectable meals! I always wanted to help her in the kitchen, but she gently refocused my attention to some other task, as the pet I played with the day before often served as our dinner the following night. I always liked being with Alba because she taught me things like balancing a basket on my head, how to hang a stalk of bananas so they ripened evenly, and how to wash clothes in the river while taking a swim. She was beautiful, warm, wise . . . And, at 18 years of age, an orphan for 8 years. So when my father questioned her about stealing money from our food allowance, I would gladly have taken the blame myself to protect her. When he threatened to dismiss her, I decided to put myself on the line by faking the theft. In the middle of the night, as I crept into the kitchen in my new role as thief, I saw Alba outside giving food to a group of children who had gathered by the fence. From what I could see, there were 20, perhaps more, children extending eager hands for a chance to eat the food we had designated as garbage. For children, they were ever so quiet.

The next morning, I practiced a small speech to present before his honor, my father, to exonerate Alba. Even as a child of 10, I knew she was more honorable in her intentions than anyone I had ever met. So I prepared for the worst by telling my father that Alba had been using the grocery money to help feed orphans. It was a moment I'll never forget as I saw my father's face turn red, and his eyes fill with tears, and his body heave a deep breath. I had seen that look before—minus the tears—and that look never ended well. His loud voice thundered as he called for Alba. I tried desperately to dissuade him from firing her and to convince him I was mistaken in what I had told him. His words resonate with me still. "Alba can't save these children by herself. She needs our help." In what seemed like an instant, my father, with Alba's help, created an orphanage and funded it for five years, after which the funding was picked up by a religious organization. While Alba remained with us for a few months after that day, she devoted the rest of her short life to feeding and caring for the orphan children.

The years that followed this event saw world changes, the biggest for me of which was the Vietnam War. It seems that either boys went to war and returned in body bags or they moved to Canada and never returned at all. My dresses got shorter, my hair grew longer; I attended sit-ins and nonviolent rallies, and I shaved my head in ninth grade to protest the war. When my father shook his head and asked why, I smiled and said, "Well, dad, the boys can't end this war by themselves. They need our help." And as he smiled, I knew he approved of the lesson he taught me when I was 10: Everything and everyone needs help to grow and change. Thus I entered into another stage of transformation from child to adult.

TRANSFORMATION FROM CHILD TO ADULT

The '70s found me ready to explore life as, what I thought then, an adult. I spent time in Spain and jumped in and out of Morocco. The Vietnam War came to an end, for most purposes, in the early '70s, and discos became the rage. My hair grew back, and my hemlines got longer. The perm and power suit fitted women with the outward tools to play in a man's world. Shoulder pads and high heels were quite a combination, as they expressed our roles as both feminine and masculine. The Ayatollah of Iran was killing young women for the very thing American females were flaunting: independence. Gasoline was rationed, and relationships began and ended during those long lines at the gas pump. *Star Wars* made its debut in 1977, as I made my debut as a high school graduate from East High School in Pueblo, Colorado. By 1977 I met a hulking young man 10 years my senior and light years my wiser, and within 45 days made him my husband.

The rest of the '70s and the first part of the '80s brought dramatic changes for me. No longer was I able to bounce from place to place, since I was now a wife and mother of two children. Although I cherished the time with my children and never failed to give them my undivided attention, I determined it was time for me to return to school. Thus I began the next transformation—from wife and mother to student.

TRANSFORMATION FROM WIFE/MOTHER TO STUDENT

My husband and I were so poor that I paid for my first semester— $60.00—with money I earned from selling my children's old clothes and toys. As my husband, Joe, was just finishing graduate school, our family of four survived on a combination of the garden the boys and I put out back and help from my parents. But relatively soon after graduation, Joe secured a job nearby, which allowed me to finish my first 2 years of college. Then, we were off to Seattle, where my husband began working as an engineer for Boeing.

The '80s were a time of change for both of us. As the Berlin Wall came down in 1989, so did many stocks; and as air traffic controllers were fired by Reagan, the industry changed, then airplane production changed, which changed engineering, which changed us. To ensure stability for our family, Joe and I decided to transform together from employees to entrepreneurs as we incorporated an engineering firm. Thus we traveled to Florida as energetic young entrepreneurs, and as business increased and the two boys grew, I completed my goal of acquiring a bachelor's degree. The '80s swiftly passed without much fanfare; on the other hand, the '90s were not so gentle. It was during the '90s that I made yet another momentous transformation—from student to advocate.

TRANSFORMATION FROM STUDENT TO ADVOCATE

In 1994, our family was privileged to welcome its fifth member, Jordan Christopher. Our then 14- and 17-year old sons—once they recovered from the shock—became phenomenal brothers, and thus Jordan entered into a family who awaited his every smile and accomplishment—even when neither smile nor accomplishment appeared.

When our child, Jordan, was 2½ years old, he was diagnosed with autism. After a painful process of testing and diagnosing, the finality broke our hearts. Not knowing much about autism, we relied on what we did know: that autism was mental retardation. As a result, we quickly began posturing ourselves for challenges that would no doubt arise. We entered Jordan immediately into therapies, and as a family we enrolled at the University of North Carolina to participate in the T.E.A.C.H.H. program. T.E.A.C.H.H. is a training program in which all teachers in North Carolina are required to enroll. For over 30 years, North Carolina has been researching and implementing teaching strategies to help autistic children. In fact, it is the only state in the nation whose state government directly supports the research and that has an intact program to help autistic children complete a college education. While its system is by no means perfect, it informed us about Jordan's education, the IEP [individualized education program], what we could and could not expect from schools, and how to proceed once we returned to Florida.

Feeling confident in our abilities to help Jordan progress as a valuable citizen, we excitedly entered him into school, as we had our other two children. Within a very short time, however, we discovered that Jordan's academic experiences were going to be very different from those of our other children. Our attempts to receive services outlined in Jordan's IEP were ignored; accommodations included in his IEP were not being made. As my child's fiercest advocate, I could no longer be a soccer mom on the sidelines. I had to take a tough stance and transform into a source of knowledge and vehicle for change. Within 2 years, I entered USF [University of South Florida] and completed an M.A. in English Education, procured a teaching position in Citrus County, and moved Jordan into a new school, where he received all the services to which he was entitled. Additionally, the Citrus County School District invested money and time into training teachers about autism. In fact, there is now an autism specialist in the district as a resource for parents and teachers. As refreshing as the change was, more challenges were ahead of us.

In 2002, Florida law mandated that any third-grade child with low reading scores (Level 1) is retained. From the moment Jordan entered his new school in Citrus County, he made tremendous progress. Concurrently, his initial diagnosis of autism had been revised to reflect a diagnosis of Asperger syndrome, which is still a form of autism but much less severe. We were overjoyed to know that Jordan could enjoy the same experiences our other children experienced—and perhaps even more because of the opportunities available to him. However, first Jordan was required to take the FCAT [Florida Comprehensive Assessment Test] and pass with a score of 3 or better. His teachers believed he would do well on the test, as he was a good reader who demonstrated excellent vocabulary and comprehension. Therefore, it was a great surprise when he received a 1 on FCAT Reading and thus failed third grade. Because there was a discrepancy between Jordan's ability and his performance on the FCAT, **I readied myself for what would become the battle of my life**.

On June 2, 2003, I contacted the Florida Department of Education about seeing Jordan's test results with more specific explanations attached. In 2003, very little information was provided about the test or its results. Because of Jordan's particular disability, it was important to know how to proceed with remediation, not to mention that the FCAT score was inconsistent with his abilities. In response to my inquiry, I received a canned e-mail that only vaguely addressed the issues I had questioned. Most of the response was vague and circuitous. For example:

> The Individuals with Disabilities Act (IDEA) states that the education of students with disabilities can be made more effective by having high expectations and ensuring their access to the general curriculum as appropriate.

As I reviewed the canned e-mail, I realized that they had not even bothered to insert Jordan's name, but rather referred to him as "your son" in the spaces provided for his name. Interestingly, this e-mail was later referenced by the Department's attorney, Nathan Adams, as including a list of "permissible accommodations and good cause exemptions" although no such list was attached to the referenced e-mail.

Unsatisfied at that time with answers provided by the Department of Education, I continued to request a manually graded test, since Jordan's performance on the FCAT test was incongruent with his abilities and performance in the classroom. On October 16, 2003, Cornelia Orr, the then Director of Assessment and School Performance, Accountability, Research, and Measurement, responded, stating "A request to rescore a student's test, based solely on a lack of a few missing points, is not necessarily a valid reason for rescoring." After nearly 4 months of unsatisfactory discussions with the Department of Education, I filed suit on October 21, 2003, for access and permission to review my son's third-grade FCAT test.

One of the more audacious events during the suit entailed a discussion with Victoria Wagner, the State Program Specialist Supervisor for K–12 Assessment at that time. In Mr. Adam's letter, dated November 10, 2003, he suggested that I contact Ms. Wagner to determine "permissible accommodation for your son." Following through on the request, I called Ms. Wagner the next day to discuss my son's situation. During the conversation, Ms. Wagner noted that she had little knowledge about ESE [exceptional student education] accommodations and that she would need to confer with an ESE specialist. In fact, as summarized in a letter I sent to her, she stated that she believed "the test questions could be restated for Jordan should the syntax of the question pose a problem for him." I offered to convene a conference call to include the ESE district specialist for Citrus County, as well as Jordan's teachers, principal, and ESE director, and Ms. Wagner readily accepted. Additionally, I invited various legislators to participate who entertained an interest in FCAT issues. Arrangements were made, and I notified Ms. Wagner of the date. The next day, November 21, I received a certified letter from the State's attorney notifying me that

> the Department is not agreeable to delay the filing to hold a conference call with legislators. Under any circumstances, the Department is not agreeable to participate in a conference call with you and others on December 3 at 4:00 P.M.

On the same day, November 21, 2003, I received the list of test accommodations that the attorney referenced in his letter of November 24. However, he mistakenly identified the accommodations as being included in a different letter written by a different person. By December 10, the Department of Education filed suit against me for attorneys' fees and costs, a threat they made on November 10 when stating:

> The Department of Education will file a Motion to Dismiss and request attorney's fees and costs . . . unless you dismiss your Complaint beforehand.

While my case won in the lower courts, it lost on appeals. Nonetheless, it received media attention and exposed the ineptitude and callousness of the agency appointed to protect children like my son, Jordan. Through this process, however, I gained allies who likewise understand the negative effects of high-stakes testing. In 2003, I became involved with Florida Coalition for Assessment Reform (FCAR) and now serve on its board. As a result of this affiliation, I have become more aware of children negatively affected by testing not only in the State of Florida but nationwide.

As a direct result of my lawsuit and involvement with the grassroots organization FCAR, there is a dialogue about transparency in high-stakes testing. FCAR and its members continue to press the State for transparency of the test, especially for children who are being retained or denied a diploma. People, including legislators, who in the past believed high-stakes tests were an effective gauge of student learning are now beginning to question the purposes of high-stakes testing and the insanity that surrounds its continued practice. Through my experiences in 2003, and through the support and alliance of FCAR, I determined that there was much more work to do in improving education. Therefore, I have recently begun another transformation: from advocate to critical theorist.

ADVOCATE TO CRITICAL THEORIST

Transformations are powerful actions not to be made lightly or without thoughtful consideration. As I transition into the years more often designated for retirement, travel, and carefree living, I am compelled to use the time to help others. As Joe Kincheloe states, "All things are a part of a larger interactive dynamics, interrelationships that provide meaning when brought to the analytical table" (2007, p. 39). We are, in essence, all connected to education. To be living is to learn; to share is to teach. Thus we are involved in a never-ending process of educating ourselves and others. In this process, we have the power and responsibility to make visible what seems at first invisible and to make possible what at first seems impossible.

Critical pedagogy is a way of looking at the life and the world in which we live as opportunities to extend generosity and trust to those around us with the intent of sharing and reaping goodness. To do this, we "question deep-seated assumptions and myths that legitimate the most archaic and disempowering social practices" (Giroux, 2006, p. 1), we attempt to "create conditions within which people can think for themselves" (Leistyna, 2007, p. 117), and we continue to "demonstrate on a regular basis that one size fits few, and there are multiple ways of knowing our world" (Janesick, 2007b, p. 243).

Thus, as I embark on this journey at this time in my life, I am prompted to recall the words of Optimus Prime: "Transformers, they're more than meets the eye." Just as Megatron and his conspiring decepticons dangerously walk among us undetected, so there are destructive practices operating among us about which we must be constantly aware. As educators, we are reminded by Henry Giroux that we must

> define [ourselves] less as narrow specialists, classroom managers, or mouthpieces for corporate culture than as engaged public intellectuals willing to address those economic, political, and social problems that must be overcome if both young people and adults are going to take seriously the future that opens up rather than closes down the promises of a viable and substantive democracy. (2006, p. 249)

Therefore, as I continue to learn more about the world in which I live—the world in which my children must live—I will continue to transform into whatever form necessary as I await my call to action.

∽

Clearly here you see that a journal may serve a researcher well. For this researcher, writing down clearly the thoughts going on in her mind as she described herself and her transformations assisted in defining her as the researcher she was becoming. When she talks of her personal activism on behalf of her son and her previous multinational life, she is on the cusp of something. It will be a few years before her dissertation is completed, but the seeds of these descriptions may be part of her own description of her role as a researcher in her eventual research project. She has established a habit of writing on a regular basis to get into the rhythm of writing. Most qualitative researchers include a description of the role of the researcher, which includes their beliefs, values, biases, and intent in doing the study. Oral historians would be well served by including such a description in any of their analysis and interpretation segments of a given oral history. It is a strong and durable technique.

Following is another stream-of-consciousness journal entry from an oral history of women leaving teaching. The writer also writes on a regular basis. Both writers begin to identify their transitions through getting it all down on paper in the form of the researcher's reflexive journal. As the next writer puts it, How can I interpret the lives of others without writing about my own life first?

CASE III.2.

ᘓᘓ

Response to a Question on the Transition from Teaching in the Public Schools to Becoming a University Professor

BY TARA H. HOLM

> You have flown away
> Here I must stay
> Walk straight with head held high
> And I will think of you
> Every step of the way.
> —LILLIE HUMPHREY, Arapaho

I knew the exact moment it happened. Tonight is a big invited performance for my 160-member honor choir. About 1,500 people would be in attendance. Everything is set up and in place. I dash home with only 45 minutes to shower and change into my black velvet director's outfit, with white lace blouse and red silk cummerbund. I suddenly stop. It's not here. I have been a performer since beginning classical piano at the age of 4 and completing that training with my first doctorate in music at age 25. The thrill of a performance is that extra adrenaline that I always draw on to both calm me and add a particular edge to the evening.

But this evening, as I look in the mirror, I know this part of my life is suddenly over. Curiously, I have little idea what this means. I hear the voices of my grandmother and my mother whisper, "Imagine where they go, for it is time to walk on." I watch myself through the performance because my interaction with the choir and with the audience comes from a different place. With the final chords of John Rutter's *Requiem*, this junior high choir from the "other side of town" is again praised with another standing ovation. I step away and to the side, I watch the kids as they bow, and I look to the back of the room at their parents. The rewards are always written in the lives of the students and of their families, never in the transience of applause, no matter how momentarily sincere.

Late that cold, crisp December night, I sat bundled up in a warm blanket on the back patio of my home and I watched the night chase the moon across the sky. I didn't quite know how things were to change, but I knew it was time to leave this haven I had called home on the edge of the prairie. I knew simply that I was a teacher, ready for new land-scapes. I sat through that night and so clearly remembered my growing-up years on the south side of Chicago, living next to the railroad tracks with only an alley separating our house from the rumble of the trains next to potters' field. The boxcars and the switchyards offered refuge for a ragtag stream of men who found their way in the late 1940s and early '50s to our back door, clutching their belongings in red bandannas and wearing tattered hats, ragged clothes, shoes that were tied on their feet, and dreams that were long ago abandoned. "Work for a meal?" I remembered their asking. "Wash up in the spigot on the other side of the house," they were told. Gram and Mom would cook them scrambled eggs, gravy, bacon, and a biscuit, and then they'd be gone, the empty tin left on the back porch swing. No one was turned away, ever, no matter how little we had. "Watch and listen," my grandmother would say. "Say nothing," my mom would gently whisper. Later, those same men would be asleep behind a tombstone, an empty bottle in a rumpled brown bag clutched in a dirty hand.

So often in those years we would walk down the tracks, picking asparagus. Mom would ask, "Where do you imagine the tracks are going?" "They end at that point. I can see it," I'd say excitedly. "No, they go on far past where you can see. You must imagine. The things in your life that will be the most valuable, you will not be able to see. You must dream, envision them, and work for them to come true. But do not let them own you." I was but 3, then 4, and although I don't think I fully understood, I remember these times so clearly. Each spring as the cottonwood flew across the back alley, I could hear the words of my mother, "You must imagine. You must dream, but you must not let your dreams own you. What you cannot see is the most valuable." And each time we walked down the railroad tracks, we would together spin stories about where we thought the tracks were going.

At morning's dawn, I had once again joined what my elders, my mother, and my grandmother and their people had called the spirit path, the journey each life takes when it seeks the purpose for which it was created. It was now time again, at the edge of the prairie, to look beyond the horizon point to a new destination, for all that had looked so familiar the previous morning assumed a distant dimension. I watched myself move through my day, and for the next 2 weeks I ended each day at the library, reading voraciously, trying to catch up on some of what had happened in the literature during the years I had spent working, learning, teaching, sharing my life with junior high students and their families. We had created all sorts of programs; taken trips to Europe with the kids every other year; started a food pantry and clothes closet open to everyone in town (that usually my families would have benefited from but now ran), which had grown immensely; developed a Parent Empowerment Project [to which] we were told no one would come [but] 80–100 parents came once a month; had all-night dance-a-thons and raised four busloads of canned goods for the homeless shelters; and gave over $9,000 a year in money the choir raised from fund raising to local charities in town. All on "that side of town," where they said it could never be done; yet it was not my doing. It was all of us working together. But now, it was time to leave. I had done everything I had come to do and more. After my first doctorate, I knew myself well enough to know I was too young to stay at the university. I needed to be connected more richly and more fundamentally to something much deeper—I needed a community. It was what I found those 28 years in public school, particularly there in Kansas.

Now, at this juncture in my readings, I found, in Kansas, the work of a woman who would become my mentor in the fullest sense of the word. Challenging her to help me shape a second doctorate, I could then return to higher education to prepare teachers of the future. We launched on an adventure that extended well beyond those 3 glorious years of doctoral studies. The day I defended my second dissertation, this one born of the passion for my students and the fight against the ways the institutions of society continued to marginalize and disenfranchise them, all the while condemning them, I booked a ticket for my first job interview. Two weeks later, I hopped a plane and found myself in a different world. I knew no one in Michigan. After 20 years in Kansas, I knew nearly everyone. Yet I felt a peace, a quiet assurance taught me by my elders, that this was the place I was supposed to be. So despite other interviews and other offers, I listened again to my personal guides, as I had that night before the mirror.

When word leaked out that I was leaving Kansas for Michigan, students' and families' expressions of love were overwhelming. At the last concert, people came, as well as sent flowers, from all over the country. Why would I leave all of this? I believe it was because it had all become too comfortable, too easy, too familiar, and too predictable. And, too, I was older. I had built all my programs on my energy, my enthusiasm, my commitment, and the time I was willing to spend with the kids. It was taking more energy to do now what had come so naturally even 10 years ago. I reasoned the kids about whom I cared so deeply deserved that person, the person who could give them so much more than I could now give.

Too, there was a whole part of me I had not used during this time. It was time for me to step back, to let go. Selfishly, it was not easy. In truth, I never thought I would care about students as much as I did about these junior high kids. I was soon to find out how wrong I was. As I sat in my den amid all the boxes prepared for moving, I excitedly opened the package that my new institution had sent, which was the suggested textbook for the first course. But as I read, I started making notes on pages. This wasn't the classroom I recognized, the classroom where young people struggled to make sense of a world that cared little about them, a world that just across the street from the school encouraged them to make in a day more money than I was making in a year, a world where they still held out hope for a future, though fragile and tenuous. This wasn't the classroom where joy and laughter could create magical learning moments, where students' daily lived experiences could help them interpret their literature books and rewrite their vacuous history books. I looked at a text filled with terms for lessons I had never heard of, though I had taught those lessons. Yet there were no young people in those pages. This was complicated by the fact that the text was written by the people in the program area who had hired me. The department I work in is so large (51 full-time faculty and over 40 part-time faculty) that we are divided into program areas, mine being curriculum and instruction.

My first experience as a faculty member of my new institution was interesting, not unusual, unfortunately. Following the opening faculty meeting, our program area met. The first item of business was a discussion about who was going to get a new office computer. "Well," said one outspoken colleague, "Tara's getting a really nice one. Do you know why?" Without missing a beat he answered his own question: "Because she's an Indian." Simultaneously everyone turned to the back of the room, looked at me in silence, slowly turned back to their agenda, and moved to the next item of business. At the end of the meeting, I said it was nice meeting everyone, as well.

Beyond that, the recollections of that first year are rekindled each time I see that glazed look in the eyes of new professors. I never minimize it, for in many ways I asked first-year questions I had never thought to ask, and without a mentor I would have struggled. I held such lofty goals of being a scholar ready to translate the stories of 28 years in the classroom into the foundation for research and the backdrop for preparing young professionals to enter into the reality of the urban classroom. I had plans for middle-grade academies, summer programs, institutes, camps, curricular designs of various kinds, programs to work with local and state urban middle schools, foundation work. And then I was told I needed to be quiet, not do anything, and get to know people for a year or so. When I asked if there were any rules of deportment, conduct, or departmental interaction, I was told there weren't any rules. Again, I talked to my elders, and they said "listen to what is not said, for there lies the truth." As I watched others trying to navigate the political reefs of no-rules, I saw they did not successfully arrive at new possibilities for themselves or for their program areas. The contradiction between being invited to come and be a part of a faculty, then being distanced by what is said and what is done, by the tension between junior and senior faculty, is an interesting dilemma.

Because our institution places a high premium on teaching and the preparation of teachers, my frame of experience was both my strength and my momentary impediment. In public school the end of our teaching year came in May, but here there was no end. One year simply ran into another. And the mail came from everywhere, no longer from just the main office. How did I know what was important? I covertly watched as older faculty sorted their mail while standing at their mailboxes. I squirreled mine away to my office, and painstakingly sorted it piece by piece, once a month following each faculty meeting, hoping I hadn't discarded something of value. Usually there were two or three big projects planned for the school year; however, in higher education we move from one major project to another, sometimes even working simultaneously on curriculum development and paper presentations while doing grant proposals. This was indeed a shift in gears.

The biggest issue as a new professor was grading. What was a "usual" master's paper? All I had ever known was what I had done. Was it the case that 50 resources in the bibliography for a midterm research paper was typical? Somehow I had never paid any attention to what my classmates had written. I had no idea what average was, only what I expected of myself. And when my students asked if I were going to use the same text the following semester, thereby enabling them to sell their books, the notion of a graduate student selling books was beyond my comprehension. A call to my mentor was a crash course in Reality 101.

Then there was the candy store for professors. The opportunities for grants, presentations, collaborative work in the program area and across college, conference proposals, foundation work, and school partnerships were the very least of all the choices. I wanted to do everything. How did I choose? But then once a month, when a college newsletter listed colleagues' work, my excitement was only exceeded by the familiar nagging: "Why am I not doing more?" Perhaps one of the most uneven personal challenges was the lack of community that still resonates with me. The constancy of seeing the same colleagues every day for an entire school year is quite a change compared to the unevenness of being with different groups who may come in only when they teach (e.g., Monday–Wednesday group, Tuesday–Thursday group, or only graduate classes in the evening). I missed the consistency of the professional community.

That first year, when I walked the floors late into the night or sat on the back patio and ate bags of M&Ms, what was it that I questioned? What was it that I doubted? It was not my decision to leave, for each new play in the theater of my life is written with familiar lines and acts from preceding dramas. Neither was it my choice of universities. That I have always celebrated. It was the reminiscent doubt of self. After teaching junior high students for 20 years, could I shift gears and teach adults? Who were these young men and women? Did I possess the skills, the passion, and the enthusiasm to ignite their own ambition? Did I have the capacity to change in the ways necessary? Could I, as Kahlil Gibran says, lead my students to the threshold of their own minds, to discover their own visions?

My mother, my elders, and my faith have taught me it is not enough to dream. I must awaken from my dreams and realize the vision that is my very life. I have joined that for which I have been created and have resisted moments of chasing the wind. It was not change for its sake alone that I sought. It was Solomon's wisdom that Hemingway wrote of to know the time for everything under the heaven, to hear answers when you know not even the questions, but are yet willing to seek. All the questions that form the self-doubt and stories of my elders regenerate me.

"Walk straight with head held high," wrote my grandmother to me as I left home, the first of my people to attend college. I have learned that means to listen more, perhaps through life's lessons of physical vulnerability and being confronted with the frailty of life. Perhaps because **in these twelve years of higher education** I have worked with the most dedicated, supportive, caring, and talented colleagues I could ever imagine. With a changing of the guard, no longer do we speak in competitive terms or in junior–senior faculty. Together we have crafted a space where we write together and think together, where our ideas benefit our students, where we provoke each other to expand our own ideas and awake us from our dreams to realize our own collective hopes. Perhaps through the stories my mother has always shared.

She never gave advice in those moments of discouragement or of joy. It was always a story, for she knew they connected me to something much larger than the moment. They connected me to that yearning to know who I was before the person I am now that dwarfed the minute conflict or elation of the moment. She would simply tell the story and then quietly move on. Advanced Alzheimer's has slowly stolen most of my mom from me. But this past December we were sitting together on the living room couch and I was reading a newspaper article to her. She had been relatively unnoticing of anything around her, essentially uncommunicative, when suddenly she reached out her frail, bony, yet gentle hand and took hold of mine. She slowly turned to me and said in the familiar cadence I remember from my childhood, "Where do you imagine they go?" I stopped reading and looked in Mom's eyes. I heard the distant whistle of a train.

Within this performance exercise of journal writing, other performance exercises may be created, such as creating poetry from the text. Poetry may also be created to record the thoughts of the reader and/or prospective oral historian or to find the symbolic language of the narrator, as well as her meaning. Poetry is endowed with strength and durability. Throughout history we have numerous examples of the use of poetry to tell someone's story. To use a few examples, the *Iliad*, the *Odyssey*, and the *Aeneid* were the collections of all the stories, folktales, and centuries of history told in poetry. In my attempt to describe a portion of the reinvention of oral history, I would like to discuss the importance and value of using poetry to tell someone's story.

USING POETRY IN ORAL HISTORY
TO REPRESENT SOMEONE'S STORY

One form that may enrich an oral history narrative or any qualitative project is the form of poetry constructed from the data. Some writers call these "found data poems." These are poems constructed by the participants in a study and/or the researcher from the data at hand, including the transcripts of the interviews, journal entries, documents, and photographs. One might say that from the moment we are born, we collect a trail of documents to signify part of who we are. We start with a birth certificate, social security card, driver's license, marriage licenses, divorce records, dental records, medical records, retirement records, and so on. We continue in life collecting documents such as mementos and cards or document our own history on video. Poring through these documents to describe, explain, and interpret another person's lived experiences is often enhanced with the use of the poetic. I encourage the use of found data poems to prompt new ways of thinking about the data and of representing the data in order to tell a more powerful and cohesive story. Likewise, interview transcripts are a good source of poetry in any form: haiku, verse, free verse, and so forth. People often ask me why I use poetry. I can only say that I think poetry helps me to make sense of the world. Poetry allows me and others, I assume, to come to some kind of meaning of events in life, or at least try. We may not get to that meaning or understanding, but we take some comfort in knowing that we are trying. Poetry also opens up the imagination and helps me in the habit of writing.

Found Data Poems in the Transcripts and Other Documents

Found data poems can be a useful and helpful technique for making sense of oral history data. In addition to selecting sections of the transcript to punctuate the meaning of the person's life, one may use any documents or journal entries as part of the dataset in which data poems can be found. Recall for a moment the example of Leona's story earlier in the book (Case I.1 in Part I). From the opening narrative, we see Leona in bed at over 400 pounds, depressed and inchoate. At the end of the narrative, through education and one key person who inspired her to take a class, a radical change took place. Notice the three examples of poetry inspired by those data in the form of haiku, free verse, and rhyme. Haiku, a Japanese art and literary form, is traditionally defined as 17 syllables long, although in translation it may be a few syllables shorter or longer.

Poems Inspired by Leona's Story and the Opening Words of Her Story

∽

Every journey has a beginning, and—although I didn't realize it back then—my journey toward becoming an educator began the day I awoke to realize that I was trapped in a deathbed of my own making, hopeless, alone, and just waiting to die. At 450 pounds I had become extremely depressed, lonely, and isolated. I spent most of my days lazing in bed, watching TV and eating junk food. At the time, I was living in seclusion in a small trailer on an isolated stretch of land on a Pacific Northwest mountain range. My doctors told me that the various health problems I had (e.g., asthma, diabetes, hypertension) were directly related to my morbid obesity. And although I faithfully consumed the medicines they administered to me, I had very little faith in their ability to sustain my life.

Haiku Example

Serendipity made me whole
Before I could object
Just in time.

Free-Verse Example

Why did I forget myself?
How did I allow this?
What made the difference?
Who changed me?
Where did I go right?

Rhyme Example

See me, see me
Fat today

Looking, looking
Far away
Changing, changing
Once or twice
Life is like the toss of dice.

By writing poetry from the data, one has an alternative mode of representing the meaning of the data, possibly to use to introduce the story or narrative components of the story or to enhance its meaning and interpretation. Poetry is one of my favorite literary tropes, and it can easily be valuable to the oral historian. In writing up a narrative of a person's life story, using poetry at the beginning to introduce the story and possibly at the end to embellish its meaning, along with interspersing poetry within the text, may be a way to force a more reflexive turn in the narrative writing process.

For another example, recall Alex's interview with Miss Humphrey (Case II.5 in Part II) and his subsequent reflections on race. Here are three found data poems from both the interview and his reflections. See how poetry is used to capture and interpret a portion of her life.

Poems Inspired by Alex's Work and His Reflections

Her active life, both past and present, has formed her sense of knowing. This takes me to a third theme that stood out in the interview: race relations. Although she was kind enough to agree to this interview and to discuss the topic of my choice, I sensed she was grateful for the interruptions. I also sometimes felt patronized by some of her comments. She said racism doesn't exist anymore, and her tone, during parts of our conversation, seemed to question my purpose for resurrecting what her words suggested she believes is a dead or nonissue. She seemed to imply that I was smarter than that. I also sensed the conversation dredged up memories she'd rather forget, including the death of her mother and father and her own racist past and behaviors. While I believe she is unduly critical of Black people, I also believe she believes Black students are smart. She thinks they make bad choices. She never considers the lessons she and others failed to teach as a possible reason for the bad decision making.

Haiku Example

Black and white
Words so tiny
Yet so colossal
Make us change today.

Free-Verse Example

Miss Humphrey, what a story
Wish you told me more.
Miss Humphrey, you gave me pain
When I asked for truth.
Your life made me choose description
To unravel this depiction.

Rhyme Example

White and black
Took me back
To a time forgotten
Black and White
Made me fight
For illusions often
Voices black
Voices white
When do they arrive?
Voices white
Voices black
How do we survive?

ɔ

From these six examples, we see how it is possible to use poetry in ways that are creative and imaginative while sticking close to what appears in transcripts and narrative reflections, as well as any documents that are provided in a study. Many say they cannot write poetry; however, even those who protest too much are surprised to find that not only can they write poetry, but they write profound and entirely thought-provoking poetry. Thus we do not abandon the transcript; instead, we use it in a new way, to reinvent oral history as a potentially meaningful and artistic endeavor.

CASE III.3.
~

Excerpts from an Oral History Transcript of 36-Year Veteran Teacher Dan Rawls, Who Also Is a Mentor to New Teachers

The following excerpts appear in the interview with Dan Rawls discussed in Case III.5.

I believe that good cooperating teachers and mentors are born. Great ones are trained. And the essence of what I am as a cooperating teacher is part of me as a human being. . . .

I honestly and truly believe that the type of person that you are is the best raw material you can start with. If you're the type of person who is judgmental, who probably expects other people to be able to do things better than you can do them yourself, who is demanding, who is unyielding, then I don't believe you will be a good cooperating teacher. . . .

I believe that cooperating teachers are responsible for creating a community of learners, and I try to build that atmosphere into my role as a cooperating teacher. I don't know everything. You certainly don't know everything. But we can figure it out together. I might know how to find out. I might know how to think about it a little better than you; that's only by virtue of age and experience. We'll work it out together.

I . . . don't recall any aspect of the training telling me or helping me be aware of what to do with a cooperating teacher, or how to help a cooperating teacher whose lesson falls flat on its face, and they're devastated because they've spent hours and hours preparing it. I don't recall any aspect of the training teaching me how to help [student] teachers learn to do several things at the same time, multitasking, listening to questions from the students, taking attendance, writing out passes, getting the lesson started, all of the different things that teachers do fairly automatically without thinking about it. Young teachers, who've never had to deal with it, have to learn how to do it, and it's difficult and it takes time. It takes time and it takes repetition. But they don't know that, so they need someone to gently guide them through. Don't let them give up. . . .

There are so many levels and aspects of mentoring. I don't understand how any teacher who has a fairly successful record cannot be a mentor on some level. But I find that most teachers, probably not all, but most teachers are natural-born mentors. They want to help when they can. We are helping kinds of people. That's part of our personality that brings us to the profession or helps make us successful in the profession. So I think that it's a natural flow of what we do each day that we mentor. We know that there's formal and informal [mentoring], there's official and unofficial, there's technical and alternative, but in some sense of the word *mentoring*, each of us mentors all the time. I believe that mentoring is as critical to . . . it's . . . it's as inherent in teachers as helping a sick person is to a doctor, regardless of the situation. If the need is there, you automatically know it, and you automatically deal with it if you can. . . .

So before I judge or before I can come down as a cooperating teacher I have to consider what it would be like for me in that same situation. Fresh out of school, lots of ideas, lots of theories, but no application to hook them to. So I am very good at considering what it's like for them. If I were in their shoes, what would it be like for me? That allows me or forces me to back off a little bit and consider the situation before I react in a way that would do more damage than good. . . .

My original intent was to help him, but I'm terribly afraid that it didn't work that way because it was not a good way to handle the situation, and what made me think about it was something made me wonder how I would feel if someone had done that to me in my absence. I think that's a critical issue for professional teachers. I think Atticus Finch in *To Kill a Mockingbird* teaches his children not to criticize people until they have "walked a mile in someone else's moccasins." I think that is a very valid argument for professional development in our encounters with administrative staff, clerical staff, custodial staff, colleagues, and particularly students. Before we jump into any problem-solving situation, we have to stop and carefully think, if we can, as much as possible, from the perspective of the other person. When you do that, the number of times that you are justified in jumping in and cleaning house, as it were, are going to be terribly, terribly, terribly reduced when you start looking at things from the other person's point of view a little bit more.

ↄ∾

As you look at these sections of the transcript, try to create your own poem to represent the meaning of Dan the narrator. One example of a found poem in this transcript to convey meaning follows:

Walking in Your Moccasins

Walking in your moccasins
Gives me pause
I understand you better now.

Thus you can see that poetry found in the contents of the transcripts offers numerous opportunities for drawing your reader into the text through poetry. It is one creative way to represent the data, that is, the words of your narrator. Another possibility for representing the data in the story is through the use of digital techniques such as photographs or videos on the websites many use today, such as YouTube. In fact, the website *www.animoto.com* is a good starting place for the oral historian who wishes to practice making a video of still photos or of an interview. Some of the features of this site follow.

- Animoto is a Web application that allows you to create video clips using graphics that are in .jpg or .gif format.
- 30-second video clips are free, or you can pay an annual fee ($30.00) and make video clips of any length.
- You upload your images, add some text (optional), select your music, and Animoto does the rest.

Any educators who teach online may wish to try this set of techniques with which students can create their own videos.

Likewise, the site *www.voicethread.com* allows your interview to be archived on the Web and shared with anyone who logs into the site. This is called "voice thread" because the site allows group conversations about any topic. All this is done with no software to install. This is a multimedia site that stores photographs, videos, documents, images, and voices. You may also create artwork and drawings on this site if your computer is so equipped. Students and teachers alike may find this site useful for taking part in document-ing history. Teachers may find this site valuable as a teaching tool, and students may use it as an outlet for their creativity. The site was originally designed for students who use Facebook, Second Life (with their own or multiple avatars), and MP3 players that can also accommodate DVDs; then it grew beyond expectations. The Voice Thread site designers note that they wish to inspire collaboration through the use of creativity—say, in a classroom or among a group of individuals—to comment on what is uploaded to the site. You may create your own account, which is free; however, there are sections for educators and business personnel who may wish to pay a fee for additional features. In any event, the creativity alone makes this site worth exploring. It could easily be a useful tool for oral historians and other qualitative researchers.

THE POTENTIAL AND ELOQUENCE
OF THE NARRATIVE IN DIGITAL STORYTELLING

In addition to poetry, digital technology is a way to tell stories. It makes sense to use the audio and video digital devices open to oral historians. I agree with Frisch (2008) that oral history is now ready for a postdocumentary sensibility. By this he means that we are able to move beyond our how-to-do-oral history, nuts-and-bolts approaches toward a deeper and nuanced interpretation of our data, so that the "raw" collection is not just sitting on a shelf. Audio and video indexing today allows us to search and access data in a new way, a richer way, so to speak. He describes the new approaches to publication and public access, for example, in this way:

> Implicit in this approach are whole new modes of publication and public access. Imagine, for example, the value of producing broadly distributed collections of richly mapped and thoroughly searchable

interviews, music, and performance or other field documentation, in which users may find and make their own meanings. In producing such a documentary source, authorship would reside not in fixed path making, but rather in the richness and openness of the map coordinates, codes, and finding tools offered to users. (p. 237)

For me and others, digital storytelling is a good way to do this. And, in fact, this is already being done. Digital storytelling uses digital photography, digital video, and many sites on the World Wide Web to tell a story about some component of our life history. Why do we tell our stories? Why do we want to hear the stories of others? Why is the narrative so powerful for us? Humankind has been involved in storytelling throughout history. Whether we rely on the oral tradition, cave carvings, the written or spoken word, artwork, danced stories, or YouTube, storytelling has captured us.

The potential of the narrative to make us feel and empathize with others is one of the main strengths of storytelling. The narrative is a way for oral historians to capture and reflect on our cultural values, our beliefs, and how we interpret the world. If Emerson is correct that all history boils down to biography, do we then all have the biographical or the autobiographical impulse? Let's assume this is a good place to start. Oral historians are in a marvelous and strong position to be master storytellers and narrative writers. We are already committed to capturing someone's story, so we are almost there. Not only that, we live in a time in which digital storytelling is an ongoing activity on the Web. Just a brief perusal of digital storytelling websites reveals nearly a million sites alone on this topic, complete with video and audio individual stories. Digital storytelling is simple storytelling in digital format. It is a deeply democratic approach to storytelling, because all age groups may have access to digital stories. If someone does not have a computer, he or she still may access these stories at their local library. Many groups and individuals are dedicated storytellers, and they offer many teaching tools and rules of thumb for the digital storyteller. Likewise, new texts are being written on visual methodologies and digital history (Cohen & Rosenzweig, 2006; Rose, 2007). Just a few main sites of the hundreds listed on the Web are given in the following list of centers; they also feature links to other sites.

SELECTED WEB RESOURCES
FOR DIGITAL STORYTELLING AND HISTORY

The following websites are rich with information and model digital stories. This list is not meant to cover everything on the Web that is concerned with digital storytelling and history, but it is a good start and most likely will lead you on a road to discovery.

www.storycenter.org (Center for Digital Storytelling)

This center, based in Berkeley, California, is dedicated to the art of personal storytelling. The Center offers workshops, programs, and services, and all are focused on capturing personal voice and facilitating teaching methods. Their motto is **listen deeply, tell stories.**

storiesforchange.net (Stories for Change)

This site is an online meeting place for community digital storytelling and advocates for social change. Multiple recorded stories are available. Recently the stories included a meeting of two granduncles who teach a young Vietnamese American about war and family and also the story of a woman who became a teacher in Boston due to the injustice she observed in schools. Social justice themes of race, class, and gender are part of the stories here.

www.eldrbarry.net (Effective Storytelling)

This site is a resource for digital storytellers with suggestions for writing a good story and examples of good stories. Multiple resources are listed and posted on a regular basis.

www.oraltradition.org (Center for Studies in Oral Tradition)

storytelling.concordia.ca (Center for Oral History and Digital Storytelling Concordia University)

www.ihtp.cnrs.fr (French Institut d'Histoire du Temps Present)

www.besthistorysites.com (Best History Sites)

This is an award-winning site that covers all areas of history, from prehistory to postmodern times. It has a lengthy section of sites on oral history, as well. This is an excellent site when you start to use the Web as a digital storytelling technique for your work as an oral historian and qualitative researcher. This site lists over 1,000 websites and links to thousands of quality lesson plans for teaching history to K–12 students, including history teacher guides and archives. There are also links to games and puzzles. The oral history section includes general resources and selected oral history projects and lesson plans. Among the many websites already listed in this book, this site adds the Library of Congress and, of course, the British Library. The oral history projects are many and varied, including oral histories of the Vietnam War, the civil rights movement, the assassinations of Martin Luther King, Jr., and Robert Kennedy, slave narratives, veterans' groups, immigrant oral histories, and one titled, "What did you do during the war, Grandma?"

historicalthinkingmatters.org (Historical Thinking Matters)

Although this website is focused on key topics in U.S. history, it may help teachers in other disciplines, as well. For example, when teaching about a time period, say, the 1770s, one may adapt some of the critical thinking activities to many interdisciplinary questions. What were business and industry like then? Who were the writers of the time? What kind of artwork was being done at the time? There are resources here for instructors and a wealth of information on getting young people to think historically. It is a prize-winning site and was created by collaboration between two historians, one at George Mason University and one at Stanford University. This site is for both students and teachers. The creators of the site approach history by presenting conflicting firsthand accounts of a historic event.

These are only some of the well-situated sites for learning about digital storytelling and that display examples of various stories from students, veterans, nurses, farmworkers, and many more community members. The clinical fields, such as medicine, nursing, and hospice care, also have availed themselves of oral history on the Web. Various agencies and professions, in fact, have created digital stories on the Web for easy access and for learning from the story. They refer to these stories as teaching tools. Other digital media include videos posted on YouTube. Many of my students post their stories on YouTube, Facebook, and MySpace, as well as making use of the blogosphere. This is the next frontier in oral history, and, like dance and choreography, it requires practice. One word of warning: Many sites change addresses from time to time, so be aware of the changeable nature of the Web. However, with persistence, you can find the site you were looking for, even if the name and address are changed. Likewise, as a historian yourself working in these media, you will have to continually upgrade your computer and software. It is one of the by-products of the digital age. Technology is constantly accelerating its forms and facets.

INTERNET INQUIRY, THE WIKI WORLD, AND COPYLEFT AGREEMENTS FOR ORAL HISTORIANS AND QUALITATIVE RESEARCHERS

This generation of Web users is using the Web for news, for developing written communication, for shopping, for meeting people, and for banking, to name a few purposes. Why should we not make use of the resource of Internet inquiry as oral historians? This is a powerful tool for developing a sense of history, reflecting on our stories, and understanding our communities in their contexts. In fact, a new generation of scholarship is developing around the Internet, known simply as Internet inquiry. Also, an international network of Internet researchers founded a professional organization in the late 1990s known as the Association of Internet Researchers (AoIR). This is a remarkable opportunity for oral historians who wish to go beyond just posting a story on YouTube, for example. The website, which explains more fully all the activities of the AoIR, is *http://www.aoir.org*. It is here that you will find newsletters, conference information, publications, a code of ethics for those using the Internet to do research, and a wiki. You need not be a member of AoIR to post on this multidisciplinary site, which explores the cultural and social meaning of the Web. For researchers, it is a well-stocked resource that grows in content daily.

Anyone can contribute to a wiki on the Web. *Wiki* comes from the Hawaiian word for "fast" or "quick." Wikis are a type of Web technology that enables anyone to modify an existing Web page. It is associated with the fast-growing and quickly burgeoning Web encyclopedia, Wikipedia (*www.wikipedia.org*). In addition, wikis are used throughout cyberspace. Wiki entries or pages are part of the **free speech movement** on the Internet. It is critical for all of us as qualitative researchers, oral historians, and citizens to learn the language and potential of creating wikis about our work.

The wiki movement originated in the hacker community, with the goal of providing free software on the Web. Hence, the use of and contributions to Wikipedia are free, that is, at no cost. But the subtext also concerns free speech. Why should it cost us something to post a story on the Web? A wiki creator would say it should not, and in fact it does not, because the Wikipedia is licensed under the GNU (GNU's Not Unix) Free Documentation License (GFDL), created by Richard M. Stallman and the Free Software Association, which basically allows anyone to freely modify a text on the Web. This is known in the wiki world as a "copyleft" agreement, to move away from and go beyond traditional individual copyrights. Many other wikis operate under the copyleft agreement. Copyleft is essentially a way to make a program free and to require that all modifications to the text are free, as well. So, to use an example, if a person finds something on Wikipedia that needs updating and corrects it, that material is also free. This only makes sense, as it more effectively uses copyright laws to allow more rights for users, say, in the area of modifying texts. What is intriguing to me as a researcher are the nuances of the wiki world in terms of underscoring the democratic nature of the Web and the implication that knowledge should be available to all for free. There is a kind of creativity with words, such as *new* and *gnu*, and a noteworthy use of the imagination in the descriptor "copyleft." A copyleft license in effect locks in various content materials. No money is exchanged. One underlying premise of the copyleft agreement is that all knowledge that is old becomes new again and that no one individual can claim ownership of it. Isn't it ironic that the newest of technologies seems to validate and take to the maximum the age-old adage that in fact there is nothing new under the sun? We might think of contributing to a wiki as volunteering to work on a knowledge base in multiple disciplines. Wikis are collaborative in nature and can be traced back in history to the concept of encyclopedias. The original notion behind creating encyclopedias was to make abundant knowledge available at a certain price. Where is knowledge more abundant than in the wiki world? All this is to say that qualitative researchers, and in particular, oral historians may find a great tool for opening their work to the world. Wikipedia and other wikis are on the Web in multiple languages and venues. It is a tool for dissemination of any amount of knowledge and is a great place for stories. To learn more about copyleft agreements and free software, go to *www.gnu.org.*

FINDING MODELS OF DIGITAL ORAL HISTORY
USING TOOLS OF THE WEB

We have at our disposal a great deal of information and variable techniques to construct and write up an oral history. In this electronic age, the oral historian and the qualitative researcher have to decide which audience to write for, in what genre to write, and whether to make the oral history available for free. I think that after these decisions are made, the age-old research techniques come into play, and the write-up of the oral history evolves into the story to be told. Let us review four examples of the powerful oral histories available to anyone in digital archives on the Web that were created as a result of a major trauma. Oral histories of Holocaust survivors, of victims who testified at the South African Truth and Reconciliation Commission (TRC), of survivors of the terrorist attacks of 9/11, and of survivors of Hurricane Katrina are remarkable. What all four of these examples have in common is that they counteract the selective amnesia so often associated with all of these events. They also bring to mind many social justice questions, such as inequality, racism, class difference, gender issues, poverty, and struggle. Let us look at some of the resource examples, all of which are available on the Web in four categories of digital and/or audio oral history: the Holocaust; truth commissions, specifically South Africa and the TRC; 9/11 stories; and Hurricane Katrina oral histories.

Holocaust Testimonies

The collection of the United States Holocaust Memorial Museum (*ushmm.org/research/collections/oralhistory*) is most likely one of the largest collections and most diverse resources for testimonies of Holocaust survivors at present. This collection has over 9,000 audio and video interviews. Researchers, students, the general public, and any interested parties can see and hear these accounts firsthand. These archives also contain the testimony of perpetrators of the Holocaust. The museum has a permanent collection of edited segments, as well as complete sets of testimonials, available. To work on the Web, you will need to get a password and sign in online for the exhibitions and the data. This rich database includes interviews with survivors of the Holocaust and Nazi persecutions, including Jews, Roma, Polish Gentiles, Jehovah's Witnesses, homosexuals, political prisoners, collaborators, rescuers, liberators, and relief workers. Interviews include testimony from individuals in Belarus, Czech Republic, Estonia, France, Germany, Greece, Israel, Latvia, Lithuania, Macedonia, Moldova, the Netherlands, Poland, Romania, Ukraine, the former Yugoslavia, and the United States. In fact, the oral history branch of the museum has completed a publication of a reference tool that is available for those interested in oral history titled Oral History Interview Guidelines. Also at this site and at the museum is the Steven Spielberg film and video archive, which includes archival film footage documenting the Holocaust and World War II. The numerous universities in the United States that house Holocaust archives can also be found through links on this site, such as Understanding the Holocaust through the George Mason University Project, to use just one example. Furthermore, the British Library, known to be the foremost and largest research center on earth, has a Voices of the Holocaust collection, along with teacher's guides and classroom activities, at *www.bl.uk/learning/histcitizen/voices*.

Other well-known Holocaust archives can be found at the University of Michigan, the Georgia Institute of Technology, the University of Chicago, and the well-known Shoah Foundation Institute at the University of Southern California (USC), as well as dozens of other sites. It is at USC that Steven Spielberg's eyewitness accounts are preserved on film.

Truth Commissions

In addition to the actual website of the Truth and Reconciliation Commission (TRC) of South Africa, many other archives hold truth commissions' testimonies. One example is the United States Institute of Peace (*www.usip.org*). Here you will find a comprehensive digital collection of truth commissions worldwide. These archives include the testimony and oral histories of individuals in more than 25 countries as diverse as Argentina, El Salvador, Nepal, Serbia, Sri Lanka, and South Africa. To use just one example, the South African TRC was set up in 1995 to investigate the human rights violations during the apartheid era, between 1960 and 1994. Archbishop Desmond Tutu chaired this committee of 17 members. Hearings were held in a public forum, a first for truth commissions. Usually these types of commissions were convened behind closed doors with a veil of secrecy. Many commissions, such as the one in Chile, gave a blanket amnesty to perpetrators. In South Africa there was no general amnesty. The applicant had to make an individual application and give testimony. An independent panel had to decide whether or not the conditions were met for amnesty. It was felt that blanket amnesty would contribute to a national kind of amnesia and that ultimately the record would be lost, thus victimizing a second time all those wounded by apartheid. Memories of all the travesties were critical and had to be recorded. An applicant for amnesty had to give full disclosure, verify behaviors, and accept responsibility for what was done. Victims had the right to oppose the amnesty with evidence but could not veto amnesty if amnesty was granted by the commission. In addition, victims were to receive a specified amount of money as reparation. The public hearings recorded violations on both sides of the apartheid struggle. Amnesty applications came from all sides, and out of the 7,113 petitioners for amnesty, 5,392 people were refused. One of the solid resources on the South African TRC is the video archive at the Yale University Law School. This videotape collection is available in 91 episodes at *www.law.yale.edu/ trc/view-_all _requests.asp.* Each episode provides detailed testimony on all aspects of the hearings, ethical and legal questions included. Specific massacres and bombings are described. Also included are testimony on torture and all justifications recited in the court hearings. It is a full-bodied picture of the impact of the TRC in South Africa. It also is a fine example of how video can be used effectively as an oral history technique. It shows how to go beyond documentary evidence. Of course, we start with the documentary evidence, but now we are ready to move forward past the documentary to the postdocumentary stage.

9/11 Oral History Collections on the Web

A remarkable collection of oral histories is available for anyone to read and think about from the testimonials of New York City firefighters, police, and first responders. Individuals who were at Ground Zero and the Pentagon were interviewed almost immediately and subsequently throughout the first year following the 9/11 attacks. It took almost 4 years to fight to make the documents public. Finally in August of 2005, thousands of pages of individual oral histories were released, and they can now be read on the Web. In the following year, 2006, an additional set of oral histories was made public, and doubtless many more will follow in additional books on this event. The immediacy of the firsthand accounts is stunning, as are their clarity, specificity, and authenticity. Some of the sections have been redacted, which was required as a compromise so that the oral histories could be made public. Here is a good example of democracy in action. The fight to disclose the information was a healing act, as well as an informational act. The knowledge of the firsthand events makes one pause and reflect on their meaning, as is the case with oral history in general, particularly following traumatic events. These stories are part of the fabric of our collective cultural history. I think that as oral historians we have an appetite for understanding, and these data help us to understand the individual event with a bit more precision, transparency, and honesty. There are literally more than 15,000 websites on the 9/11 oral histories alone. One can type in the words *9/11 oral histories firefighters*, for example, into Google and wade through the amazing data collections. There are additional sites for police officers, first responders, and eyewitnesses. Key providers of food and beverages and the clergy are also interviewed. As oral historians we are able to record in print, audio, and video the stories of our time. YouTube also has lengthy and numerous collections of oral history interviews on the aftermath of 9/11. This is an amazing resource for historians and other researchers.

Hurricane Katrina Oral History Projects

Another traumatic event of our time was Hurricane Katrina, which broke the levees of New Orleans, causing havoc, death, and destruction. Harvard Medical School has an oral history site with testimonials from individuals who lived through and experienced Katrina from the first announcements of the hurricane to the present (*www.*

hurricanekatrina.med.harvard.edu/oralhistories.php). It is an archive that helps us understand the lived experience of persons in the context of social inequities and the side effects of poverty.

Another site on Katrina oral history is Do You Know What It Means? (*www.doyouknowwhatitmeans.org*). This site takes its name from the signature Louis Armstrong song, "Do You Know What It Means to Miss New Orleans?" Here there are stories, photographs, and videos that capture the events and personal memories of one-time residents now displaced, as well as individuals who returned to New Orleans.

Both sites are designed to help all of us understand life before, during, and after Katrina. Do You Know What It Means? focuses on survival. This song has also been used on YouTube as the background for a video of scenes from New Orleans immediately following the hurricane.

These examples are just some among the vast store of archives and individual audio or video recordings of persons' lives available for review and reflection. Each offers us data on major events in our history. Many of my students ask me why they should care about something that happened in the 1940s or even the recent event of Hurricane Katrina. I try to use that question as a teachable moment to open a conversation on historical and critical thinking. What else do we have but history to make us more aware of the present circumstances? Santayana's famous and often quoted statement could never be more apt. I can only agree with him that if we do not learn something from the mistakes of history, we are condemned to repeating those mistakes.

AWARENESS OF ETHICAL AND LEGAL ISSUES

Doing oral history means that we follow the ethical guidelines of our professional organizations and treat all of our participants with respect for the truth and authenticity of the story being told. Without a doubt, all qualitative researchers, and especially oral historians, deal with ethical issues by virtue of working with real people in real settings face-to-face. Ethical issues may arise in field work, and as they do, we deal with them. We explain them in the context of our reports and try to be facilitators, brokers of agreement, and watchdogs of the profession. The current controversy between various institutions and IRBs regarding whether or not oral history research should come under the jurisdiction of IRBs is still unresolved. In fact, *www.institutionalreviewblog.com* is a blog on which researchers can discuss the ethical issues surrounding IRB approval. A recent blog posting indicates that a growing number of universities are removing most oral history research from IRB jurisdiction. The following excerpt, retrieved from *www.institutionreviewblog.com/2009-04-01-archive.html*, discusses the University of Missouri—Kansas City's (UMKC) **respectful oral history policy**. (The extracts in Case III.4 are taken from UMKC's policy statement.)

CASE III.4.

ᐁ

Blog Posting on Respectful Oral History Policy

BY ZACHARY M. SCHRAG

The policy has a number of elements that set it apart from the typical university policy, which seeks to cram oral history into a system designed for medical experimentation. Instead, it adapts only those elements of the medical IRB system that encourage historians to follow their own discipline's ethics and best practices. . . . UMKC understands this. Its policy notes that

> In keeping with the public role of an historian in a democratic society, these responsibilities, especially when conducting narrative interviews, can necessitate a confrontational style of critical inquiry. So while historians do not set out to hurt their interviewees, oral historians are expected to ask tough questions in their interrogation of the past. . . .
>
> After reviewing these resources on their own, the researcher is strongly encouraged to discuss their research protocol with peers before implementing their research protocol. In some cases, peer review by members of one's own department would be most useful; in other cases, a researcher might be better served by seeking review from a colleague in a different department.
>
> To foster these kinds of conversations among the faculty, the Social Sciences IRB Subcommittee for Oral History will hold two meetings per

semester . . . to discuss "Best Practices" in oral history. Faculty experts in oral history will guide these conversations. . . . These meetings are designed to meet the needs of researchers seeking advice and peer review for their research protocols. They are also designed to meet the needs of Chairs and/or designees interested in learning how to advise researchers in their departments to make responsible decisions regarding oral history. . . .

UMKC takes seriously the carefully negotiated 2003 agreement between the American Historical Association and the Oral History Association and OHRP [Office for Human Research Protections], even posting a copy on its website.

The bottom line is that the researcher makes these determinations in careful consultation with the Chair of the department or another official designee appropriate to the kind of study being planned. Together this determination is based on shared understanding of all relevant guidelines and their shared expertise in their specialized field of scholarship.
—POSTED BY ZACHARY M. SCHRAG, 11:26 P.M., APRIL 25, 2009

The author then describes respect for the IRB and mentions that UMKC joins other universities, which include **Amherst College, Columbia University, the University of Michigan, Ann Arbor, and the University of Nebraska, Lincoln**, in adopting the OHRP's decision to remove oral history research from IRB jurisdiction.

This is the dialogue that continues online and in our hallways. As an oral historian, it is critical to find out what your institution requires and work through each case accordingly. Beginning researchers doing a dissertation, for example, are generally required to fill out an IRB form for oral history projects, even given the federal regulations (see Appendices F and G). I require all my doctoral students to go through the IRB process, as we are in a public field, education, that falls under numerous accrediting agencies and guidelines. I imagine that this dialogue and debate will continue as more and more people become aware of what their home institutions require. This is one ethical issue that will be sustained. The movement from outside review by an IRB to review by one's own peers has merit, and some universities are beginning to act on this idea.

Legal as well as ethical guidelines are part of the fabric of oral history. A good tool for understanding the legal rules and implications thereof can be found in *Oral History and the Law* by John A. Neuenschwander (2002). This resource contains a great deal of information in its 93 pages and includes basic release forms and contract forms (see Appendix E). Also explained are issues regarding privacy, contracts, deeds, gifts, copyright, and ownership and transfer should you be working with an archive at an institution, for example. Now with the increasing use and coverage of Internet storage spaces and with the AoIR ethical guidelines in place, much research has shifted to the digital mode. Regardless of whether we use digital storage or traditional archives, oral historians must pay attention to legal, as well as ethical, issues. In addition, other types of ethical issues arise from time to time, as they do in any qualitative project, depending on the case in question. For example, Blee (1993) studied women of the Ku Klux Klan and described the ethical problems with being unable to reach mutual agreement with her interviewees regarding their memories of the Klan. Her article described the tension she as an oral historian experienced between her responsibility to her interviewees and her responsibility to her profession and to society. In any event, as ethical issues arise, we, as qualitative researchers and specifically as oral historians, describe them and try to explain them for the reader.

PUTTING SOME PIECES TOGETHER: CRAFTING AN ORAL HISTORY REPORT

To help you think about how to write the report of an oral history project, see the following case example from a recent methods course, which follows the techniques we use. The writer selected someone to interview based on his experience in the area, found themes in the transcripts, and made sense of these in his analysis. Martin M. Morris interviewed Dan Rawls about how he mentors student teachers into the profession. An excerpt from this interview was used earlier in this portion of the book to show the researcher's journal entry and a poem created from the study. This example indicates the flow and movement of the interviews and the reflection on the interviews by the researcher. The researcher also discusses the processes he experienced in doing this oral history project.

CASE III.5.

꙳

Interviewing a Master Teacher and Making Sense of It

BY MARTIN M. MORRIS

INTRODUCTION (EDITED)

What follows is a shortened version of a class assignment. The doctoral student, himself a practicing high school teacher, interviewed a master teacher who has been teaching for 36 years. Both are in English Education as doctoral students, as well. The topic of the interview was focused on the master teacher's role as a cooperating teacher (CT). In the field of education, beginning teachers are placed in a master teacher's class to practice teaching. This is called "student teaching" and is often referred to as "preservice teaching." Student teaching is considered the capstone experience. Thus it is important that an individual be placed in a class with a dedicated, experienced master teacher. In this case, the teacher has been teaching at the high school level in Tampa, Florida, since moving from a small town outside of Albany, New York, in 1986. He is in his late 50s and has been host to a full-time student teacher at least 10 times during his career and opened his classroom to a multitude of preservice teachers who were looking to observe a true master.

In my first interview with Dan Rawls, he said that one of his greatest sources of professional pride is the fact "that almost half of my interns of the past have become teachers in my school, and all of them are still there." This is quite a testament to his ability to mentor preservice teachers and truly engage them in the work of the profession on a long-term scale.

For this paper, my desire was to interview a master teacher. I also wanted to practice doing transcripts, analyzing chunks of data, practice coding data, and come up with a model of what occurred in this practice life history interview project.

THE CRITICAL RELATIONSHIP

The field experience should be a time of teacher growth, where a strong correlation is built between the theoretical foundations established during teacher preparation and the practice of teaching. Field experience should offer preservice teachers a chance to experience a nearly vertical learning curve. It is critical that a clear understanding of the potential impact of the cooperating teacher be understood so that those who undertake this responsibility can be taught to take advantage of their ability to enhance the learning relationship they share with their student teacher. Without this constant push by the cooperating teacher, the student teacher will not be prepared to enter their own classroom.

Cooperating teachers can learn to take advantage of the student-teacher internship as a time of practice, reflection, and experimentation. Cooperating teachers spend time encouraging growth and reflection in the development of their craft. Clearly, one of the most powerful ways that classroom teachers can contribute to the profession is to become a cooperating teacher and mentor, and becoming a good mentor is not as easy as it seems. So what is it that makes Dan Rawls so adept at helping fledgling teachers become successful teachers? One way to find out is to ask him.

INTERVIEWING AS A RESEARCH TOOL

For this particular class project and for an examination of the role of the cooperating teacher, an interview with a master cooperating teacher seems especially appropriate. As someone who has studied the role of the cooperating teacher in the past and been a cooperating teacher four times, I decided that a semistructured interview would be appropriate.

Since I was hoping to learn more about Dan's views of his position as a cooperating teacher, I used a responsive interviewing model (Rubin & Rubin, 2005). This model is about "obtaining the interviewee's interpretations of their experiences and their understandings of the world in which they work and live" (p. 36) while being grounded in interpretive constructionist philosophy. This philosophy says that in the construction of meaning between the conversational partners, the partners critically impact what is learned in the process of the investigation. The findings from this interaction understand that the truth that is discovered is but one truth that could be interpreted differently by another observer. This philosophy is appropriately fitting because the conversational partners form a relationship during this interaction, and this must be considered when interpreting information discovered during the interaction. For the purpose of this paper, two interviews will be conducted. The initial interview questions were structured in the opening-the-locks pattern suggested in Rubin and Rubin (2005). The opening-the-locks interview pattern is structured around a small number of main questions intended to allow the conversational partner to talk at length (Rubin & Rubin, 2005). This is my intention in the first interview: to let the master speak.

FIRST INTERVIEW

1. What does your work as a cooperating teacher mean to you? Why do you feel that this work, which is voluntary, is worth doing?

2. Becoming a cooperating teacher requires that you take an additional training in clinical education through the school district. Discuss how this training prepared you to be an effective cooperating teacher. What were the strengths and weaknesses of the training?

3. Discuss any other training, either formal or informal, that has helped you in your role as a cooperating teacher.

4. Can you describe, in as much detail as possible, what a typical day as a cooperating teacher looks like?

5. Tell what you like/dislike about your role as a cooperating teacher.

6. What do you need the university, the school district, and the teacher's union to do to make your job as a cooperating teacher more successful and more productive?

PREPARING FOR THE INTERVIEW

To prepare for the interview, I gathered my Olympus DS-2 digital audio recorder, two copies of my first interview protocol questions, and my notebook for field notes. I tested the recorder in advance several times to make sure the recorder was working properly and that the sound was clear. I also had an extra pack of fresh AAA batteries, though the battery indicator on the LCD screen of the recorder indicated that the batteries were nearly full strength. Interview questions were provided in advance.

Dan and I have known each other for several years as teachers working for the school district of Hillsborough County (Tampa), Florida, and more recently we have become better acquainted as doctoral students. I know that Dan has served as a cooperating teacher (CT) many times, has done extensive reading on and training in the areas of being a cooperating teacher and more specifically in mentoring, so I believe he has sufficient expertise to answer questions about the role of the cooperating teacher and how to improve the effectiveness of this role.

CONDUCTING THE INTERVIEW

The first interview lasted from 3:55 until about 5:10 P.M. During the interview I allowed my conversational partner to talk at length and only followed up with probes when I immediately saw a need to ask more. I also made notes during the interview about themes that I thought might prompt questions during the second interview and that might give me ideas for follow-up questions and prompts during the initial interview. I am a strong believer in choosing my conversational partner wisely. If someone with great knowledge and expertise is available, then it is critical for me as the interviewer to minimize my involvement in the discussion (Rubin & Rubin, 2005) lest I interfere or unduly influence what is discovered. Dan is a tremendous person to interview because of his vast knowledge of his subject matter, his deep convictions about the profession of education, his ability to clearly explain himself, and his unmatched experience as a cooperating teacher.

TRANSCRIPTION AND CODING

Due to my busy schedule and personal obligations, I did not transcribe the interview until 2 days later. While I would have preferred to do this sooner, I still believe that I was able to capture the essence of the interview accurately because it had gone so splendidly and was still quite fresh in my mind and because of the high quality of the audio recording. Once the transcription was done, the important part of the process began. The analyzing of the first interview forced me to look for themes that arose that piqued my interest and seemed important to my conversational partner. Since this was an interview with only one follow-up interview to come, it is impossible to accomplish what might be done in a bigger project, such as comparing themes across interviewees. The key to this interview was to discover themes and develop appropriate follow-up questions to learn more so the data could be reported. The next steps to examining the first transcript were to create codes for the themes and then pull out the specific quotes that spoke to those themes.

SECOND ROUND WITH THE MASTER

For convenience, we met in the same place as the first interview, only a month later. Again, I arrived early. Several questions are constructed in the second interview to offer my conversational partner a chance to fill in information that I may have overlooked. This also may lead to the interviewee revealing what is important to them. If Dan focuses on the theme of being a reflective teacher repeatedly, then this is important to him in his role as a host teacher. The questions added to the interview for this purpose are:

1. Since we spoke last, is there anything that you thought of that you wanted to add before we begin with new questions?
2. Is there anything I should have asked that I didn't?

Questions Based on Gaps in the First Interview

There were a number of questions that presented themselves to me as I transcribed the initial meeting, as well as when I was analyzing the transcripts. While I only had one more interview left to complete the project, I included all possible questions and reordered them in order of priority to my project. If Dan brings up a different topic that he wishes to discuss, then I will follow my conversational partner down his path. The questions I added that were not necessarily based on themes found in the first interview are:

3. Can you tell about your greatest success as a CT? What made it successful?
4. Can you tell about your greatest failure as a CT? What made it a failure in your eyes?
5. How did this impact your future performance as a CT?

Questions Based on Themes

The final influence on the type of question that I created for the final interview was based on the theme and coding that I had done during analysis. I discovered three themes in the initial interview: (1) the theme of **reflection on teaching** and its importance to becoming a good teacher, (2) the role **mentoring** has on the final success of a student teacher, and (3) the theme of the **benefits and contributions** of his work. The questions that grew from these themes are:

1. What is reflection? Can you give a specific example of one time when you taught a student teacher to reflect?
2. Can you give an example of one time when you used reflection to improve yourself as a CT?
3. Tell about mentoring in your role as a cooperating teacher.

During the follow-up interview, like in the first, I listened for themes and opportunities for follow-up questions. Once the data for the second interview were transcribed, I took them through the same process as the first and looked for themes offered by my conversational partner. The next step was to write up the data of each interview, as well as offer any reflections, implications, and conclusions offered by the data.

The three themes which struck me in the first interview were used to construct most of the questions for the second interview. The themes of mentoring, reflection, and the benefit of the role of host teacher for the cooperating teacher were more deeply discussed in the second meeting, as were several questions where gaps were found in the first interview. Dan's thoughts on each of these themes, as well as a newly discovered theme of **empathy**, are illuminated in the following.

MENTORING

Dan has been a cooperating teacher many times and has read and written extensively on the topic. Because of this experience, he has a very unique perspective when discussing the role mentoring plays in the relationship between the cooperating teacher and the student teacher. One of the issues he brought up was the tremendous amount of time it takes to properly host a student teacher: "I spend a lot of time with interns when I am assigned one as a cooperating teacher." And when asked about the differences between being a cooperating teacher and being a mentor, Dan responded, "the difference I see between a mentor and being a cooperating teacher is nothing more than time on task. I always have to be on duty. Interns have my e-mail address, I always make sure that interns have my home phone number, and I always make sure that they know that if they have a meltdown in the middle of the night that they should call and talk about it." The full-time nature of this role requires that the host teacher be committed to the job.

Dan sounded off about what it takes to be a good cooperating teacher. He said that "just the desire to become a good cooperating teacher . . . is not enough. You have to have certain other characteristics and desires." He went on to say:

> I believe that good cooperating teachers and mentors are born. Great ones are trained. And the essence of what I am as a cooperating teacher is part of me as a human being.
>
> I honestly and truly believe that the type of person that you are is the best raw material you can start with. If you're the type of person who is judgmental, who probably expects other people to be able to do things better than you can do them yourself, who is demanding, who is unyielding, then I don't believe you will be a good cooperating teacher.

This focus on personality characteristics shows that Dan values cooperating teachers who are supportive, understanding, and knowledgeable. While these characteristics seem to be very sensible, they are not always considered when choosing a host for a student teacher. When asked about the responsibility of the cooperating teacher, Dan responded:

> I believe that cooperating teachers are responsible for creating a community of learners, and I try to build that atmosphere into my role as a cooperating teacher. I don't know everything. You certainly don't know everything. But we can figure it out together. I might know how to find out. I might know how to think about it a little better than you; that's only by virtue of age and experience. We'll work it out together.

As for the district training received to become a cooperating teacher, Dan said:

> I . . . don't recall any aspect of the training telling me or helping me be aware of what to do with a cooperating teacher, or how to help a coop-

erating teacher whose lesson falls flat on its face, and they're devastated because they've spent hours and hours preparing it. I don't recall any aspect of the training teaching me how to help [student] teachers learn to do several things at the same time, multitasking, listening to questions from the students, taking attendance, writing out passes, getting the lesson started, all of the different things that teachers do fairly automatically without thinking about it. Young teachers, who've never had to deal with it, have to learn how to do it, and it's difficult and it takes time. It takes time and it takes repetition. But they don't know that, so they need someone to gently guide them through. Don't let them give up.

Dan went on to describe some of the skills and modes of thinking that student teachers should gain during their practice teaching experience:

I think one of the more important ones, and there are probably many, but I think one of the more important ones that don't get enough exposure is the ability to know your limits in any given time, in any given situation. For instance, one of the attributes of a beginning teacher is that they're going to be able to solve all problems, for all kids, all the time. And they try so mightily to have the perfect lesson plans, to talk to the children in just the right way, to handle deviant behavior in just a certain way. To deal with all situations in a way that they decided at some point in the past—when they were not the teacher in the classroom, but when they were the student in the classroom—is the way to do it, perhaps based on their interpretation of theory or research, and oftentimes they become so disenchanted when they discover that things don't always work the way we think they're going to work. And I think that is critical that we help new teachers, and I don't mean to be flip about this, and don't think I'm underemphasizing it, but I think it is critical that we help new teachers learn to say "oh, well" once in a while or learn to say "I did my best and it didn't work." Or in a more general sense, we help new teachers understand that there are limits to what we can do. That doesn't mean that we shouldn't strive, that doesn't mean that we shouldn't set high standards, that doesn't mean that we shouldn't set high expectations for ourselves, our abilities, and our students, but it does mean at some point, you have to recognize that there are certain things, that despite our best efforts, and our best preparation, will not come out as anticipated. You have to learn to live with those things. . . . I like to encourage young teachers, when you get into your car this afternoon to go home, and you close the door, metaphorically close out school, and leave it here emotionally. That doesn't mean not to be reflective at home, that doesn't mean don't do lesson plans, don't do your preparations, don't think about how you can handle a situation, or how you would handle a situation better, but emotionally, leave the job at the job. All my college students have heard me say this so many times that when I start it now they finish it for me, "I would rather have a good teacher for 20 years, than a great teacher for five." I do believe that as soon as teachers recognize their own emotional limits, they will be more ready to settle for their best, followed by "oh, well."

Clearly, Dan subscribes to the idea that there comes a point when situations are beyond a teacher's locus of control. This is a difficult concept to pass along to student teachers because they enter teaching ready to save the world, and if this message is delivered less than gently, it could scar the enthusiasm of the new teacher beyond healing. This concept, while difficult to digest at first, is an important step to surviving the first few years in the teaching profession, and it appears Rawls has found an avenue to deliver this message in such a way that his student teachers stay in the profession.

To close the discussion of mentoring, Dan was asked about the difference between mentoring and being a cooperating teacher. Dan focused on how mentoring must be part of a teacher and that the ability and desire to mentor seems to be a major component in the makeup of anyone who is a decent teacher:

There are so many levels and aspects of mentoring. I don't understand how any teacher who has a fairly successful record cannot be a mentor on some level. But I find that most teachers, probably not all, but most teachers are natural-born mentors. They want to help when they can. We are helping kinds of people. That's part of our personality that brings us to the profession or helps make us successful in the profession. So I think that it's a natural flow of what we do each day that we mentor. We know that there's formal and informal [mentoring], there's official and unofficial, there's technical and alternative, but in some sense of the word *mentoring*, each of us mentors all the time. I believe that mentoring is as critical to . . . it's . . . it's as inherent in teachers as helping a sick person is to a doctor, regardless of the situation. If the need is there, you automatically know it, and you automatically deal with it if you can.

Clearly, Dan Rawls has strong beliefs about the role of mentoring when it comes to being an effective teacher and especially being a successful host to a student teacher.

EMPATHY

Throughout the interviews, Dan regularly talked about putting himself in the shoes of the new teacher, about how important it is for him to remember what he knew and what he didn't know when he was at the point of his career where his mentees are currently. For example, during the first interview, he stated:

> So before I judge or before I can come down as a cooperating teacher I have to consider what it would be like for me in that same situation. Fresh out of school, lots of ideas, lots of theories, but no application to hook them to. So I am very good at considering what it's like for them. If I were in their shoes, what would it be like for me? That allows me or forces me to back off a little bit and consider the situation before I react in a way that would do more damage than good.

Visibly, Dan has a caring and empathetic approach to how he guides his student teachers. While I did not notice this theme in the first interview, I was still able to pull out of both interviews examples of this compassionate approach to guiding new teachers into the profession. Often, student teachers are faced with a mentor who believes that it is a good idea to "toss the new teacher into the drink and see if they can swim."

> I am very opposed to cooperating teachers who believe that as soon as they can get the intern or student teacher ready, that they can walk out of the classroom and they never return again. I also believe it's a very bad idea to sit in the classroom throughout the entire student teacher's internship, because the responsibility of authority always will stay with you while you stay in the classroom. So you have to leave them their space. You have to be supervisory around the periphery. Because you have to know that they are okay, and they have to know that you're there if they need you.

In this same vein, I asked Mr. Rawls about a time he had done something that he regretted or that he felt he had not served his student teacher well. In response, he told about a time when a particular student teacher was not being especially successful, and how he tried to alleviate the problem. Dan decided that, while the student teacher attended a required meeting at the university, he would talk to the students about why they were so resistant of the intern. Upon reflecting back on the day, Dan realized he had made a terrible mistake. Through reflection and empathy, it is apparent how Dan practices what he preaches as a host teacher.

> My original intent was to help him, but I'm terribly afraid that it didn't work that way because it was not a good way to handle the situation, and what made me think about it was something made me wonder how I would feel if someone had done that to me in my absence. I think that's a critical issue for professional teachers. I think Atticus Finch in *To Kill a Mockingbird* teaches his children not to criticize people until they have "walked a mile in someone else's moccasins." I think that is a very valid argument for professional development in our encounters with administrative staff, clerical staff, custodial staff, colleagues, and particularly students. Before we jump into any problem-solving situation, we have to stop and carefully think, if we can, as much as possible, from the perspective of the other person. When you do that, the number of times that you are justified in jumping in and cleaning house, as it were, are going to be terribly, terribly, terribly reduced when you start looking at things from the other person's point of view a little bit more.

Unmistakably, Rawls understands the power of his role with student teachers and understands that young teachers "automatically see you in the knows-all, can-do-all, be-all vision. They don't want to accept that you are not going to do things for them. You're going to help them do them for themselves." This perception of the host teacher is a powerful position that must be handled carefully by those who choose to undertake this work.

A final example of Dan's empathetic approach is when he discussed a student teacher's knowledge of subject matter and especially of the literature that must be taught in the curriculum. He focused again on the perspective of the student teacher and how the host teacher must be, by nature, a supervisor of sorts, but how this position can be approached in various ways.

> So the job necessarily results in being a supervisor, expert, authority figure, and are not ones that I particularly like, but I think that they are by-products of having taught for so long, having a unique relationship with the children in my classroom, and having a vast knowledge of the content of my subject area only because I've done it for so long. Sometimes it is difficult for me to remember, when a young teacher doesn't know

who wrote a certain story, and I have to step back and think, Why do I know that? How did I know that? Did I know that at that point in my life? Probably not. After many years of experience you forget sometimes or you can forget sometimes that you had to, that you had to learn it, too. So they have to learn it. There are by-products, I think, that come with the territory.

Empathy is a quality that Dan values and emulates in his role as a cooperating teacher. He patiently employs empathy in his dealings with young teachers because it would be easy to expect them to know curriculum and how to deal with every situation and then tell them they are failures; but instead he continually places himself in the shoes of his student teachers to ensure that he is serving them in their best interests, as he considers himself at early points in his teaching career.

REFLECTION: THE SINGLE MOST CRITICAL TEACHER BEHAVIOR

Dan believes that "reflection is the single most critical teacher behavior." In terms of teacher reflection, Dan defines the practice as careful, introspective, analytical, critical review of anything that you have heard, seen, said, done, or thought during the course of your professional day. Schön (1983) described this process as one where:

> The practitioner allows himself to experience surprise, puzzlement, or confusion in a situation which he finds uncertain or unique. He reflects on the phenomenon before him, and on the prior understandings which have been implicit in his behaviour. He carries out an experiment which serves to generate both a new understanding of the phenomenon and a change in the situation. (p. 68)

This change is seen in the growth of the teacher and their ability to improve their craft on a daily basis. This constant improvement over time leads to one becoming what is often referred to as a master teacher.

One of the most telling things that Dan mentioned in our second interview pertaining to reflection and why it is important was the homespun quote that makes "a distinction between people who teach 30 years and people who will teach one year 30 times." The idea of not changing practice over the course of a career compared to constantly improving appeared to be very motivational to Dan and inspired in him a bulldog desire to ensure that he and the new teachers he influences maintain the practice of constant reflection.

Dan discussed how he introduces young teachers to the idea of reflection. He said that when student teachers are observing him in his classroom,

> if a decision I made or an action I took required or I believe that it required explanation, then I would make sure that [the intern] had that explanation because I want them to have, when they saw me make a decision maybe they would consider the decision harsh, maybe they would consider the decision impassionate or not compassionate, if there is such a word, but I want them to know that there was a rationale as to why I chose that course of action. That's how they build their repertoire of realities about actually teaching in the classroom. When you're solely responsible for the students' learning and for their behavior, it's also a good model for them so that they learn that there should be good sound rationale behind the decisions they make in the actions they take in the course of the day in regards to their student contact and their decision making regarding their lessons, so I want them to have a repertoire, a library of experiences to draw from vicariously that they've seen me go through. But I also want them to know that everything has a reason. And everything is thought out beforehand. Everybody occasionally makes mistakes, and you say I made a mistake. I shouldn't have done that that way.

One critical behavior that I see Dan exhibiting for his student teachers is his willingness to show that he is fallible. Many preservice teachers believe that they have to be perfect, and Dan immediately gives them a chance to see that the practice of teaching is [fraught] with mistakes but that the key is to reflect on them so as not to make the same mistakes over and over—to be constantly improving practice.

When Dan was asked how being a cooperating teacher impacted his day, he described the change by saying that with a student teacher:

> I feel that it's important to verbalize for them the rationale behind your decisions. Probably many days are longer, because you will have to sit and debrief with the cooperating teacher at the end of every day, as well as many debriefings throughout the course of the day. . . . This is what we are going to be doing, and this is why we're going to be doing it. This is how we are going to do it. And then at the end of the day, you go back and look at what was done, how it went, how it might need to be changed tomorrow, how it might need to be changed the next time you do it, why

it might be a good idea to throw that short story out and use a different short story for that concept. All of the thinking that we do so automatically is just verbalized. In that verbalization, that communication process takes time. So the day is probably longer and much more full of the verbalization of things that we normally keep inside and normally do automatically.

Dan considers the role of reflection the most important teacher behavior. He makes time to ensure that interns for whom he is responsible take time, with an expert, to verbally reflect on their craft on a regular basis. Because of this, he said:

> I always require interns to talk to me about their lessons and reflect on what happened during the day. I meet with interns each and every day, at the ends of periods if necessary, at the end of the day definitely, and during conference periods. I like to have interns reflect out loud for me what they did with their lesson, why they did it, and . . . how successful they feel it was in moving toward the objectives of their lesson. So one of the things that I'd like interns to do is be constantly reflective, and I truly believe that the only way a teacher can become a better teacher is through constant diligent self-reflection.

This is not a practice that Dan reserves only for new and preservice teachers. He also expects himself to reflect regularly on what he is doing in his classroom.

> Reflection is the only way to improve, in my opinion, because if you don't know something, if you don't know a fact. . . . Like I would like to know right now why we put B.C. after a date and A.D. in front of the date. I don't know that. I'm going to try and find out. A student asked me that today. I can go find out. Reflection is what makes me want to go find out. It's reflection that makes me have the strength to say to the student, you know, I don't know. I should, but I don't. That's a great question. I'll find out.
>
> It's reflection that makes me be able to say I'm going to listen to this student before I respond or before I react. It's reflection that brings me to say I want to take a course on that at the university. It's reflection that makes me go back to a student and say, "you know, John, I'm sorry I reacted that way to that situation. That was inappropriate. I was tired, I already had eight emergencies in front of you, and that was inappropriate. It was wrong, and let's deal with it differently." It's reflection that helps me know what is important, must be done in teaching, in the administration

of teaching and the paperwork. It's reflection that helps me sort out all those details of all those things I talked about. Without reflection, I would be an automaton who would be going into work at a certain time every day, going through the script, the technical aspects of being a teacher, and going home every day. It's reflection that gives me depth. I much prefer the term *educator* to teacher because I can help students learn. I can't make them learn. Reflection keeps that balance for me.

Since Dan believes that being reflective is critical to his own growth and success as a teacher, it is clear why he would so faithfully require this practice from future teachers.

One of the critical aspects of teacher preparation is encouraging reflection from teachers-to-be:

> Everybody at the college level, once the students enter their professional studies phase, which I believe is in their junior year, needs to emphasize and reemphasize and maybe even, like I do in all of the college classes that I teach, require the students to hand in reflective papers as observers, as teachers.
>
> I insist that my preservice teachers that I teach through the university write reflection papers weekly. I do not allow them to repeat to me things that they've done, things other people have done, their host teacher, their cooperating teacher, without spending a bulk of their time and effort in telling me what that experience, be it personal or vicarious, what that experience meant to them. How do they feel about the experience, whatever they observed, experienced, whatever they saw or did. I'm more interested in how they felt about the experience than I am the experience itself.
>
> Everything they do I make my students think about. . . . I believe that reflection is the single most critical teacher behavior.

Dan also believes that his constant reflection on his practice as a teacher has carried over into his role as a mentor and cooperating teacher:

> There's always an opportunity to step back and say, was that the best it could've been? Therefore, each time I get an intern to work with, or even to mentor a beginning teacher in the PNE [Practice in New English] program or am asked to assist a new teacher or a struggling teacher, I reflect on what I've done in the past and consider if that, given this situation,

and given the personality of the new teacher, everybody's different, so you can't treat any two interns the same. The kids are different. The situation is different. The time and place are different. The intern is a different person. So the impact of reflection is that I know that I've improved because of reflection as a cooperating teacher. But I also know that the next time I'm a cooperating teacher, I will do it differently, and hopefully better differently than I did the last time.

When asked how he knows that his method of teaching interns to be reflective teachers is effective in turning them into reflective teachers, Dan responded:

None of us knows, I don't believe, that anything we teach anybody is going to stick. I must say, and again, I'm not an arrogant or pompous person by nature, but I'm hoping it isn't the words that come out of my mouth that shows them the value. It's what they see in me as a person, and what they see in me as a teacher.

If they respect me, if they think I'm good at my craft, they might emulate what I do to get that way and to stay that way, and so I think modeling being a reflective teacher is most essential. Anybody can stand there and say, "now you should be a reflective teacher," but if I don't show in my daily behaviors that I am a reflective teacher, it's going to be nothing more than a different set of standards for you than it is for me.

Dan uses specific techniques to guide interns to becoming reflective. It is obvious that he has clearly defined reflection as a critical component in becoming a good teacher and that he has also thought long and hard about how to gently guide fragile new teachers to see the good and bad in their own teaching without their feeling like they are under attack. Dan said:

I verbalize my thinking. By the same token, I do the same type of thing when it's them that I'm critiquing. I say, you know, first of all, I never tell them that something didn't go well. I ask them. In true conversation and probing, I lead them to realize that the lesson didn't go well. And I always follow up essentially with, "hmmmm, I wonder why? Let's analyze it and dissect it and take it apart and look at the pieces. Maybe we don't have to change the whole thing. Maybe it's just this portion." So I guess I verbalize with them and for them what I do internally every day, all day, all the time.

I insist that my criticism, my critique, if you will, or my evaluation of student teachers' or preservice teachers' works for the classroom and how they handle lessons, the decisions they make, how they handle certain issues, how they handle classroom management, how they handle situations like late homework assignments, discipline problems, all the various things apt to come off the floor. Rather than indicate to them that what they did or said was weak or inappropriate or could have been better developed or whatever, my response to them always is, "well, think about it, let's think about it." What was the situation? How did you respond to the situation? And is it possible that there are some alternative ways, alternative responses, that might have been more effective? That might have produced a more desirable outcome? That is my usual way of talking to beginning teachers or preservice teachers to get them to think carefully about every dynamic that's happened in the course of their teaching day and if the way they handled that dynamic could have been handled in any other way that might have been more productive.

To wrap up his thoughts on how he knows that reflection becomes part of student teachers' daily routines, Dan said, "It becomes a habit after a while, it becomes a behavior that they just are doing."

THAT ONE IS MINE

An area often overlooked is the benefit that the cooperating teacher gains from the internship experience. Dan focused on several of these benefits at various points during the interview, as well as his one struggle with the role. One of the biggest benefits he saw for himself was **his ability to contribute to the profession.** He said:

[My goal is] to do whatever I can to make sure that the teaching profession, the business of teaching and learning, is left in the best possible hands. Otherwise I won't feel that I've made as much of an influence on the profession as I could have.

I really think the job of cooperating teacher means a great, great deal to me. My entire adult life, I have done nothing but work in the field of education. Now that I'm older, I'm looking forward to a pleasant retirement, doing some writing, doing some research, and doing some work with the university. But after 30-plus years in the profession, and being a person who firmly believes in the essence of public education, I'm in what I like to call my 'passing the torch' phase of my career. I don't just want to leave the business to anybody. I want to do everything I can to make sure that the profession that I have served for over 30 years is being well taken care of. One of the ways I can do that is to try to influence and affect as many young people coming into the profession as possible. Being a cooperating teacher is the vehicle that allows me to do that.

Undoubtedly, Dan is heavily invested in his role as a cooperating teacher. This investment can be seen more when examining how he believes he benefits from the position.

More of the ways he sees himself benefiting from this relationship with student teachers is in his ability to observe his own students from another perspective. Dan believes that the ability to turn over his classroom to a student teacher allows him to see his students as he has not seen them before:

> I think what I really like is being able to sit back and learn things about my students that I see from a slightly different angle than if I'm standing in front of them. I get to see their reaction to certain things differently. . . . I really respect my children. I teach in an inner-city school, an urban school that has several, that has a high minority rate and a lot of children from difficult backgrounds. . . . So my point is that one of the things that I truly enjoy about the role as cooperating teacher is watching the children develop and become functioning, responsible, decent human beings. And sometimes it is the first time that they had to do that and is the first time that they had the training and the encouragement to step themselves to look at the other person, to look at the other person's job to see how difficult it is, and to give them a chance and watch them develop and compliment them. I'm sure most of my children don't get a lot of adult supervision, but it always pleases me to see the children change, as well as how the young teacher changes.

Dan goes on to discuss how he also grows as a teacher. Interns enter his class having read different texts and sat in different classes, and he feels like he benefits as an instructor from watching preservice teachers plan and teach. Dan described one specific example of this:

> The other way that I benefit, and this is a big thing, is that I learn so much. First of all, I get new ideas. They come with all these ideas from the university, and I find them very handy. One notable example is, several years ago it was popular here for one of the professors, I think a methods professor, to have their kids do an activity called the Alligator River

Problem. And I just love the Alligator River Problem. I never had heard of it until an intern brought it to my attention. Now I use it for all kinds of things. You can use it for character discussion, you can use it for talking about personality and physical traits of characters with the students, you can use it to talk about the ethical requirements of being a friend, what is required, there are a lot of things you can do with the Alligator River Problem, and I use it every year for something or the other, and I just love it. But I must say I learned it from an intern.

While the benefits are great, the only real difficulty that Dan described as a constant struggle in his role of being a cooperating teacher was the loss of control over his classroom, the need to give up control to someone who cannot yet perform as a teacher the way he can:

I don't always like giving up my class, and it is difficult for me, and I'll admit this openly, because I figured this out through my own reflection. And I work on it constantly, but it's difficult for me not to be the authority on everything. When an intern says something that is factually incorrect, when an intern goes about using a strategy that I think is not as well executed as it could have been, when an intern handles a situation in a way that I wouldn't handle it, though they may be just as correct, I have to be careful that I don't get into, "this is the way I do it. And I do it this way, so therefore it's the only right way." And sometimes that's difficult, but that's the only thing. It really is. I don't always like giving my class up, but I work through that, and that always goes okay. And I don't always like having to staple my tongue to my upper lip so that I don't blurt out corrections. But that's about it. Other than that I enjoy the role.

While there are always going to be pitfalls to serving in this role, there was one benefit that seemed to stand out from all of the others: the idea that Dan, upon retirement, will leave behind a legacy of teachers who will serve in the same capacity as he has.

One of the most interesting things that Dan said in either of our interviews was about his mortality and how he would like to look back on his professional life:

I'd like to think that at some point in time someone's going to be looking down from on high and point out to the great decision maker of the universe, that good teachers came from me, that good teachers came from me, that good teachers came from me, and I hope I rack up some points. I really believe that I am proud of having affected the profession of education by helping good, energetic, bright young people transition from being a college student to being a professional teacher, and as I've said, to the very best of my knowledge, all of the teachers who've interned under me are still in teaching, and many of them are at my school.

Dan also has strong ideas about the qualities and characteristics that good teachers need to have to be successful. He pointed these out on several occasions during our interviews:

"Great teachers are born. Good teachers are taught in the college of education." I believe that because it is my contention that training future teachers is a critical, necessary, integral part of professional development. Training them in classroom management, training them in how to use content, training them in how to use instructional strategies, I think that's all critically important.

Dan went on to focus on the attitudinal disposition of successful teachers and said that:

The essence of what distinguishes great teachers from good teachers and maybe even good teachers from bad teachers is the type of person that goes into teacher training programs. So I just wanted to add how important I feel that there are certain personality traits, compassion, and sincerity, that you can't learn, I don't believe. You either have them or you don't. If you do have them and you go into teacher education, then the teacher training curriculum will refine your skills as a teacher, but the raw material, that I think is necessary for someone to become a great teacher, they are born with.

I asked Dan if there was one piece of advice he would pass along to preservice and new teachers that would help them benefit from his experience. To this he replied:

I believe there is one attitude or frame of mind that I try desperately to teach all younger colleagues, be they interns under my supervision, young teachers, anybody I come into contact with, actually. I have found that success, successful longevity as a teacher, requires certain attitudinal positions. It is easy, I believe, to worry overly much about the administrative staff saying one thing and doing another, or one member of the administrative staff saying one thing and another member of the administrative staff saying something different, so that you are confused and it is not helpful. . . . Sooner or later, that cancer of criticism takes on a life of its own, and you spend your day waiting to see what somebody else does that you disagree with. I think it makes for a very unhappy working situation. So if there is one thing that I think I have tried very hard to teach interns or student teachers in my care, and I think there is a wonderful phrase for it, "Don't major in minors." Figure out what you're here for and what you want to accomplish and do it. . . . So I try to teach the younger teachers not to be distracted by the many numerous and tempting, agreeably very tempting, things that go on and things that people do and things that people say, and occurrences, but to keep your priorities very, very much straight. Just go in there and do what you think you should do.

When asked about the qualities he hoped to see in the teachers and future teachers that he will point to from on high, Dan focused on one simple yet powerful practice that he hoped his former charges would exhibit:

I will want to see teachers who believe in their heart of hearts that they have something to offer young people and are willing to do whatever it takes to do just that. If it means disagreeing, and if it means going against the flow, if it means being civilly disobedient, if they honestly and truly believe that they know what is best for the children in their charge, I hope they will act according to the best interest of the children. It is, of course, important that they remain within the confines of the law, but there's nothing outside the law that they could do or say that would be in the best interest of children. But there is occasionally a policy or a rule made at a school that is not in the best interest of children. It is made in the name of expedience, efficiency, ease for someone else, in the name of control, curricular demands, and I think teachers have to be prepared and be ready, willing, and able to stand up and say, I can't in good conscience do that in my classroom, because it's not in the best interest of my children. And be able to take what comes with it for those actions. If you truly believe that what you're doing, and that what you have to offer in the way you offer it to the children is best for them, they have to be able to fight for what they believe. . . . And sometimes it takes time, it takes posturing. It takes getting on committees, it takes getting into the political arena, whatever it takes. But whenever teachers who have studied with me see this happening that is not in the best interest of the children, it is their obligation in one way or another to fight against it.

In the end, Dan found his role as a cooperating teacher significant in his larger role as a teacher and educator. He has strong, well-thought-out ideas about mentoring and reflection, as well as the benefits he receives from serving as a cooperating teacher. Also uncovered was an empathetic side to this master teacher that may hold a key to the success of other host teachers if time is taken to examine this aspect of the job. All of these discoveries could lead researchers to further study.

IMPLICATIONS AND REFLECTIONS

The process that Dan went through to become a quality cooperating teacher is not clearly revealed in this paper, but it is clear that he has a commitment to the profession, has reflected on his experience, and cares deeply about the next generation of teachers who will soon take the reins from him and lead the teaching profession into the future. Unless their cooperating teacher discovers these elements, mentioned earlier, on their own or naturally uses them when dealing with the intern, then the relationship will be in danger of failing from the start. This failure will be punctuated by the student teacher not being prepared for their future career.

REFLECTING ON THE PROCESS

Overall, I think this paper illuminates the work of one teacher who is respected for his work as a teacher and a cooperating teacher. I think it is important to listen carefully to the people who have served in this role successfully because they may have some of the answers as to how to make this a more powerful experience for preservice teachers. I feel that there are four areas where I feel I could have improved this work.

The greatest weaknesses of this paper can be found in the interviewing process. To begin, I did not do a good job of asking probing questions in the first interview. In reading the transcript, I was amazed at how I bumbled through the follow-ups. I know this is a skill that takes lots of practice, but reading the transcript of how I handled these questions has made me refocus on the importance of this skill. One of the reasons for this bumbling was my poor note taking during the first interview. I found it very difficult to concentrate on what my conversational partner was saying and jotting useful notes. The second interview I did a far better job of focusing on keeping decent notes, and this helped me formulate my follow-up questions and probes more efficiently, even though Dan spoke at length and in great detail in the second interview. I know that Rubin and Rubin (2005) believe that how a researcher takes notes is an individual characteristic. For me, I now know that I need to compel myself to do this better.

Upon reflecting on the first interview and my reading of Rubin and Rubin (2005), I decided to create a cheat sheet to help me remember to ask particular kinds of probing questions. I think this also contributed to the quality of the second interview. I thought of this much like a football coach has a card with the plays that are available for a game. They know the plays, but it is helpful to have a reference in the heat of battle.

While not a weakness, one aspect of this paper to consider is that I am an insider in several ways in the relationship with my conversational partner. Dan and I have both served many times as cooperating teachers, we have been colleagues for years, we are both doctoral students, and we are good friends. While this insider–outsider perspective is debated in the literature (Rubin & Rubin, 2005), I cannot help but think that all of this influences Dan and what he will say and not say to me. I think this is human nature. While I think the interviews went well, I also believe that this reflective process will help me do better in the future when conducting these personal interactions.

In the area of examining the data, one thing I found to be troubling was my occasional lack of attention. I sometimes found my mind wandering and would have to return to a portion of the transcript that I had already read. I realized that marking text must be done over time, giving myself breaks when needed. This is not something to plow through because it will not be done well.

In the writing I was concerned that I did not know how to write the interview sections. We had practiced interviewing in class, I read about coding and searching for themes in the book, and in class, we had looked at a sample paper, but I did not think to read the section that described the interview. Finally, and likely the strongest influence on this paper, I have very strong opinions about the importance of the role of the cooperating teacher. Since I began my doctoral program I was certain that my dissertation would focus on some aspect of the influence of the host teacher during internship. The extensive reading and writing I have done on this relationship makes it difficult for me to see where these influences might have crept into my results. I know that the questions I asked were influenced by my knowledge of the topic and my interest in particular areas of teacher education.

EXAMPLES OF THE TRANSCRIPTS (EDITED)

This is an example of an excerpt from the transcript of the first interview.

Q: All along the way, you said, you said that the difference between a cooperating teacher and a mentor was not much. What things are different about it? I just want to kind of follow up on that.

A: I suppose that there are some shades of differences. Being a mentor on any given situation might be more temporary than being a cooperating teacher is an all day, every day until the job is done. And being a mentor might be just helping somebody out as an ad hoc person when they need help as long as they know you're there. But being a cooperating teacher requires more vigilance, I believe. Requires more time. And requires more supervision. I am very opposed to cooperating teachers who believe that as soon as they can get the intern or student teacher ready, that they can walk out of the classroom and they never return again. I also believe it's a very bad idea to sit in the classroom throughout the entire student teacher's internship, because the responsibility of authority always will stay with you while you stay in the classroom. So you have to leave them their space. You have to be supervisory around the periphery. Because you have to know that they are okay, and they have to know that you're there if they need you. I always require interns to talk to me about their lessons and reflect on what happened during the day. I meet with interns each and every day, at the ends of periods if necessary, at the end of the day definitely, and during conference periods. I like to have interns reflect out loud for me what they did with their lesson, why they did it, and how they feel, how successful they feel it was in moving toward the objectives of their lesson. So one of the things that I'd like interns to do is be constantly reflective, and I truly believe that the only way a teacher can become a better teacher is through constant diligent self-reflection. I picked that up here at the university. I don't know that I've ever heard it at the school district level. So I think maybe, maybe in educational terms, the difference I see between a mentor and being a cooperating teacher is nothing more than time on task. I always have to be on duty. Interns have my e-mail address. I always make sure that interns have my home phone number, and I always make sure that they know that if they have a meltdown in the middle of the night that they should call and talk about it.

Q: So what I hear you saying is that it's more time-intensive than just mentoring. I mean, it's mentoring, but it's mentoring to the 10th power or some Nth power.

A: That's really what I believe, and I'm sure there are probably, I mean, people who are experts and have studied this for many years and read everything there is to read and done a lot of writing and thinking and teaching on it probably have some other finer distinctions, but generally I see being a cooperating teacher differing from being a mentor only in the time involved. And I can't really think of any other major difference.

Q: Can you describe in as much detail as possible what a typical day as a cooperating teacher looks like? From when you arrive at school, to your first interactions with the student teacher, even what you do to prepare before they arrive for the day, at the end of the day when, when dealing with them?

A: I don't know that I see that the day changes all that much except that your role changes, and it depends a great deal on what level the intern is at. In the very early stages, I would start my day by discussing with the intern what I was going to be doing that day, and why I was going to be doing it. Then there in the course of the day in every opportunity, if a decision I made or an action I took required or I believe that it required explanation, then I would make sure that they had that explanation because I want them to have, when they saw me make a decision maybe they would consider the decision harsh, maybe they would consider the decision impassionate or not compassionate, if there is such a word, but I want them to know that there was a rationale as to why I chose that course of action. That's how they build their repertoire of realities about actually teaching in the classroom. When you're solely responsible for the students' learning and for their behavior, it's also a good model for them so that they learn that there should be good sound rationale behind the decisions they make in the actions they take in the course of the day in regards to their student contact and their decision making regarding their lessons, so I want them to have a repertoire, a library of experiences to draw from vicariously that they've seen me go through. But I also want them to know that everything has a reason. And everything is thought out beforehand. Everybody occasionally makes mistakes, and you say I made a mistake; I shouldn't have done that that way. But there's also a rationale why it was a mistake. The answer to the question, I guess, though, about what a typical day looks like, I think, is that it doesn't look any, it doesn't look much different except, I believe, you spend a lot more time verbalizing the things that normally stay internal when you are in charge of the classroom or when you're going to always be in charge of the classroom.

I don't usually talk to people about why I do what I do. Why I teach what I teach and why I teach it the way I teach it. But with a cooperating teacher, I feel that it's important to verbalize for them the rationale behind your decisions. Probably many days are longer, because you will have to sit and debrief with the cooperating teacher at the end of every day, as well as many debriefings throughout the course of the day. The day is probably longer. You need to make time in the beginning of the day, in addition to the things you normally do in the beginning of the day, to set the interns' stage in their minds. This is what we are going to be doing, and this is why we're going to be doing it. This is how we are going to do it. And then at the end of the day, you go back and look at what was done, how it went, how it might need to be changed tomorrow, how it might need to be changed the next time you do it, why it might be a good idea to throw that short story out and use a different short story for that concept. All of the thinking that we do so automatically is just verbalized. In that verbalization, that communication process takes time. So the day is probably longer and much more full of the verbalization of things that we normally keep inside and normally do automatically. When a young teacher comes to you, they automatically see you in the knows-all, can-do-all, be-all vision. They don't want to accept that you are not going to do things for them. You're going to help them do them themselves. Sometimes it is difficult for me to remember, when a young teacher doesn't know who wrote a certain story, and I have to step back and think, Why do I know that? How did I know that? Did I know that at that point in my life? Probably not. The students are still going to see you as their teacher. The intern is going to see you as someone who never makes it a mistake, always has an answer for every problem, a solution for every problem, knows everything there is to know about the field, and that just isn't true. But we can figure it out together. I might know how to find out. I might know how to think about it a little better than you; that's only by virtue of age and experience. We'll work it out together. So I don't like, I don't like the labels of, I like the term *cooperating teacher* an awful lot better than the term that they use in New York, which I believe was *supervising teacher*. I don't like that, because I don't see myself as a supervisor. I don't see myself as an authority figure that lords over the intern. I guess there are some cooperating teachers that sit around and wait for the intern to make a mistake. But I don't like that role. I like the role of, well, let's see what happens if that doesn't work and go from there. So we do it.

Q: Can you tell what you like and dislike about your experiences as a cooperating teacher? Things that have come out of it? The worst things, the hardest things, anything along those lines?

A: I like the usual things. I like seeing a young teacher be successful. I like seeing a young teacher saying, hey, I'm gonna be all right. I chose the right profession for the right reasons. But I must admit that one of the things that tickles me more than anything else is watching the children learn to learn from another person. I really respect my children. . . . So my point is that one of the things that I truly enjoy about the role as cooperating teacher is watching the children develop and become functioning, civil, responsible, decent human beings. And sometimes it is the first time that they had to do that.

BRIEF DESCRIPTION OF HOW THE MAIN THEMES WERE CODED

I chose to code the interviews electronically using the highlighter available in Microsoft Word. The key for these codes was as follows:

Mentoring = Blue

Reflection = Green

Value of role = Yellow

Important quotes = Purple

Empathy (new theme discovered in second interview) = Red

Then I went through the transcripts color coding the areas where these were found. My next step would be to develop a model of what I found in these two interviews.

SUMMARY

In this part of the book characteristics of oral history and qualities of oral historians were discussed. The technique of keeping a researcher's reflective journal was described, and examples of journal entries were used to show evidence of the value of the researcher's reflective journal. It is a valuable tool to focus the writer and a place to keep a log of activities, problems, and issues that may arise while conducting an oral history project. Another technique in oral history projects is using poetry found in the data to represent what was found in the story of the individual under study. Examples of poetry created from the transcripts was provided. Digital storytelling was briefly discussed as another resource for oral historians and qualitative researchers. Selected websites that utilize digital storytelling were also briefly described. Digital oral history examples included the Holocaust testimonials, oral histories of 9/11 firefighters and others on the scene, survivors of Hurricane Katrina, and testimony of the TRC of South Africa. Key and ongoing legal and ethical guidelines that are part of the fabric of doing oral history and related valuable resources were addressed. A case example of an oral history interview with a mentor teacher was described and reflected on.

PERFORMANCE EXERCISES

1. Create a poem from an excerpt of a transcript. You may choose any type of poetry or a found data poem that uses only words in the text.

2. Find at least three sites on YouTube that have to do with Hurricane Katrina stories. Look for the messages in the video and find at least three themes in each, as well as themes that overlap. Write three pages on your interpretation of these themes.

3. Practice writing a journal entry as a researcher reading an excerpt from an oral history project. Write three pages of your thoughts about this piece, and create at least one poem about what you thought the narrator meant in this piece.

4. Do research to locate your discipline-based professional organization, such as the Oral History Association, and/or any other professional organization in your field to find the code of ethics of that organization. Select an organization you wish to be active in and join that organization. Most have a website with news-letters, information, job postings, code of ethics, examples of recent publications, and so forth. This is a good way to get connected in your field and to begin and maintain professional networks. Often very low rates are offered for student memberships, and they may have many benefits.

5. Write a journal entry as a dialogue with yourself about the pros and cons of IRB approval for oral history projects. What are the ethical implications? Are there also legal implications? Keep a dialogue on paper. Check out blogs on these topics. What can we learn from them?

PART IV

~

HARMONY

The Art of Making Sense of Oral History Projects with a Choreography of Social Justice

> People are hungry for stories. It's part
> of our very being. Storytelling is a form
> of history, of immortality too. It goes
> from one generation to another.
> —STUDS TERKEL

INTRODUCTION

One of the great things about doing oral history today is the fact that the historical record is inclusive. We embrace the use of oral history, as the record clearly shows, for all groups, races, and religions, as well as people involved in traumatic events, and as a result are catapulted directly into the postmodern conversation on social justice. Earlier in the book, reference was made to oral histories of Hurricane Katrina, which, of course, unmasked some serious social justice issues regarding hurricane preparedness, emergency services, poverty, race, class, gender, and, of course, life and death. Likewise, the oral histories of 9/11 survivors, first responders, and onlookers also revealed another set of social justice issues. Although social justice is mentioned in popular media and in many universities, for our purposes, in an attempt to define social justice for this book, let me say that social justice is contested territory. When one group of privileged individuals is accustomed to having their stories told, what happens when those on the margins of society raise their voices to be heard? As the changes in society globally encourage diversity due to multiculturalism and by virtue of demographics alone, one could say that we are in a period of movement toward a more equitable understanding of society. Inclusion of various and multiple competing perspectives, which oral historians and other qualitative researchers have regularly validated, described, and documented, is at the heart of the work of one who wants to understand history. Yes, there is that famous line that history is written by the victorious. Nonetheless, it is undeniable that, as a result of the civil rights movement; the feminist movement; recent movements for gay, lesbian, bisexual, and transgendered individuals' rights; and the recent election in the United States, there is a steady movement toward understanding and explaining our differences rather than assuming that one size fits all. Oral historians are at a great moment in time and at a great place on the continuum of the history of ideas. We have the tools to describe and explain firsthand the lived experiences of those involved in active social movements and social change. Furthermore, we are including more voices of persons who have never before had the opportunity to tell their stories. Race, class, and gender are active topics in my own field of education. Schools today are very different from schools of 50 or even 25 years ago. It is common to have multiple races, languages, ethnic groups, and cultures represented in public schools in urban, suburban, and rural schools. The rise of bilingual education and ESL programs and the growing awareness of students with special needs in special education programs indicates how far we have come and how far we have yet to travel. In this next section, I explain my own journey into oral history through dance and choreography as art forms. This began with my study of the writings of John Dewey on art and experience. Just as the dancer and the choreographer perform through the instrument through which life is lived, the oral historian, as research instrument, performs through the media of the written or visual narrative.

WHY I DO ORAL HISTORY

I do oral history for a number of reasons. First, it is a fit with my background in dance, choreography, and qualitative research. Second, it is one of the most user-friendly forms of research, that is, it need not be tied up in ivory-tower jargon. My students take to it readily and say that for the first time research makes sense to them. They also say they were frightened at first to even think about becoming researchers because they could not see how they could be part of the research process. They are in transition to the role of graduate student. This new role is awkward at first. Yet, oral history and, in fact, all qualitative narrative approaches are an avenue to research for them. Third, it is a method that captures storytelling at its best, something a choreographer would appreciate. Fourth, it is the method that describes how life is lived. Art and experience are folded into each other with oral history. My major influences have been John Dewey in education and Erick Hawkins in dance. One of the most profound contributions of John Dewey to our understanding of art and experience, for example, began with his book *Art as Experience* (1934). Here Dewey immediately declares that if we wish to understand the nature of art, the first thing we need to do is to forget about the art hanging in museums. He explains more fully that **we simply cannot separate the art of human experience from the experience of art**. Yet what do we see around us? We often see a watered-down revision of what we know as art within the frame of the "art world." This consists of agents, dealers, gallery promoters, sales representatives, and futurists who predict the next big fad, for example. In such an environment, the actual work of art or artifact itself is an afterthought. As a result, we start thinking of the work of art as something we hang on a wall. This may lead to forgetting the fundamental tenet that **art begins with and in some experience** of the world. For Dewey, there is no work of art apart from experience. He wrote that the physical object of art, such as a painting, a dance, or a song, is the "art product," whereas the actual work of art is what "the product does with and in experience" (1934, p. 3). Thus art is a process within a given experience. It exists within a context of a given history, culture, language, and vernacular. It is about a lived experience. Furthermore, for Dewey, creativity and vision are part of the aesthetic experience for both the artist and the spectator. Both feel and see something in the product or work of art. Dewey's *Experience and Nature* (1925) also figures into his articulation of aesthetic experience and inquiry. For Dewey and others, **experience is art.**

When Dewey discusses the intuitive quality of experience, he wants us to think about the underlying and deeper meaning of an experience. Dewey actually uses Tennyson's "Ulysses" to illustrate this point:

> Experience is the arch wherethro'
> Gleams that untravell'd world,
> Where margin fades
> Forever and forever when I move.

Dewey added then, "For although there is a bounding horizon, it moves as we move. We are never wholly free from the sense that something lies beyond" (1934, pp. 193–194). In short, Dewey is arguing that art is experience and that experience is necessary for art to be art. A work of art, or product, situates the experience for us. Dewey also speaks of aesthetics as part of experience, and *Experience and Nature* (1925) offers some insight into the topic. It is here that we find Dewey's description of experience as unified and one of a kind:

> The pervasively qualitative is not only that which binds all constituents into a whole but it is also unique; it constitutes in each situation an individual situation indivisible and unduplicable. . . . Distractions and relations are instituted within a situation; they are recurrent and repeatable in different situations. (p. 74)

In this passage and others Dewey foregrounds what he means by the value of an experience as an individual experience, which fits with ideas on contemporary choreography. It would be difficult to find a choreographer who would disagree with Dewey. Perhaps dance, of all art forms, is the clearest example of this point. For even with a choreographed dance, every performance of that dance is one of a kind, and each performance is different. Dancers' bodies exhibit differences and uniquenesses every day. One day you are stiff, one day you are fluid. One day you have a leg or arm in pain, another day you are pain free. Movement on a pain-free day looks very unlike that on a day when you have a sore or pulled muscle. For more detail on Dewey's notion of experience, see Alexander (1987). In any event, the point Dewey refers to on more than one occasion is that the nature of an experience is unique, it is whole, and it is able to be characterized aesthetically or in some way is aesthetic. If there is a product attached to the experience, such as a dance, a portrait, a painting, a film, or an oral history narrative, we are asked to remember how experience serves as the basis of art.

Dewey goes on in his writings to explain how any work of art or any experience of art "moves as we move." . . . This sense of the including whole, implicit in ordinary experiences is rendered intense within the frame of a painting or a poem" (1934, pp. 193–194). Dewey acknowledged the "exquisite intelligibility and clarity we have in the presence of an object that is experienced with aesthetic intensity" (1934, p. 195). Thus the belief that the qualities of art include the temporality or time of the artwork in history, the intensity, the understanding, the clarity, and the intelligibility of the art product is mentioned regularly in Dewey's work. This led me to evolve in my work as an educator to do work that illuminates the lived experience of an individual. Through working in public and private educational institutions and witnessing the inequities from system to system, I naturally gravitated to critical pedagogy. Critical pedagogy is an orientation very much like that of the artist. It requires that one be a critical agent as a public intellectual. As such, I question and continually negotiate the terrain between theory and practice and art and experience. The classroom is an elegant space in which one can move beyond just knowledge to understanding. Qualitative researchers, especially oral historians, have an opportunity to raise questions and document stories of the lived experience of every race, class, and gender orientation and actually attempt to understand how this may benefit society. The work of Paulo Freire in *The Pedagogy of the Oppressed* exhorted us to pay attention to marginalized groups from around the world and in our own neighborhoods. What better way to pay attention than to listen to their stories and document those stories? In my privileged place in academia, I have the opportunity to use the lived experience I have had as a dancer, choreographer, and social justice advocate to enhance my teaching of qualitative research methods.

My dance influences came from all my teachers in New York City, but most profoundly from Erick Hawkins. Hawkins founded his own school and company after working in many other major companies and with the most famous dancers in the world at the time. He was insistent on using newly created music and media in live performance. He was uncomfortable with taped music and never used it, which put him at odds with many modern dancers and choreographers. The term *modern dance* refers to the dance and form apart from ballet that evolved in reaction to the strictures of ballet. For example, the inorganic foot and leg movements that resulted in excessive injuries in ballet were just one thing modern dancers disavowed. Hawkins (1992) considered modern dance as evolving in the late 1920s, and most dance historians would agree. He explains why ballet "went down" in this way:

> The reason why it is inevitable, sitting in the seats as spectators or we as dancers, composing and dancing new dances, need the revolution, the direction called "modern dance," and the reason why it is inevitable is because the tradition of dance which grew out up in the Renaissance in Europe, which we now call ballet, is "theoretical." It is based on a concept of movement which is essentially diagrammatic and opposed to the immediate apprehended kinesthetic sense of movement. (1992, p. 23)

Hawkins saw the naturally occurring revolution in dance as paralleling what was happening in society, a change toward understanding the world, the body, and society from an organic, not a mechanistic, perspective. This is much like our current revolution into a postmodern paradigm.

Hawkins was a pioneer in many ways, like John Dewey. For example, Hawkins collaborated with the musical community and worked with many modern composers. Thus Hawkins was stressing the Dewey-like theme of collaboration and connection to a given community. Hawkins believed in the free expressive form of dance, also based on human experience. At the age of 82, Hawkins wrote the now famous *The Body is a Clear Place* (1992), which consists of chapters based on lectures given while he was artist in residence at various universities and colleges and on interviews given to various professionals on the topic of his dance and choreography. In this book, he passionately explains his philosophy of dance in action.

Erick Hawkins has been described as a true dance radical. His theory of art and dance are similar to Dewey's in more than superficial ways. Hawkins was radical because he went to the root of dance, saying that dance should be totally free movement. By this he meant dance should not separate thought and action. He believed that choreography and the resulting dance should be immediate and freed from space. He believed that dance should explore movement in and for itself. The pure fact of movement is the poetic experience of the present "now" moment. He wanted to throw away all crutches, so to speak, and find the deep physicality, intensity, and passion of the experience in the dance. He once said that, in fact, he would like to see the audience not just "look" at a dance with their eyes but with their whole bodies (Hawkins, 1992). Throughout a lifetime in dance and choreography, Hawkins tested the boundaries of our understanding of dance as experience, as art, and as a form of inquiry into both art and experience.

Hawkins believed that a teacher doesn't actually "teach" a student. Rather, a teacher allows the student to uncover basic movement principles. Ultimately, the student is the best teacher. Hawkins believed that any information that a teacher may have exists in the realm of fact and so is accessible to anyone who will seek it out. Hawkins was a student of Zen Buddhism and often used Buddhist techniques to illustrate his ideas. For example, he was fond of recalling:

> When the Ten Thousand things
> Are viewed in their oneness
> We return to the origin
> And remain where we have
> Always been.
> —SEN T'SEN

For Hawkins the student of dance should understand movement to be able to be free of movement. One way to view Hawkins's ideas about dance is to revisit his now famous January 4, 1962, response to questions posed by the editor of *Wagner College Magazine*. Hawkins was asked: "What do you consider the most beautiful dance?" (For a full text, see Hawkins, 1992.) Hawkins's response included the following statements:

1. Dance that is violent clarity.
2. Dance that is effortless.
3. Dance that lets itself happen.
4. Dance that loves the pure fact of movement.
5. Dance that does not stay in the mind, even the avant-garde mind.
6. Dance that loves gravity rather than fights it.
7. Dance that never ignores either audience or music . . . or fellow dancers.
8. Dance that is grown up.
9. Dance that reveals the dance and the dancer.
10. Dance that knows dance is and should and can be a way of saying NOW.

Thus Hawkins captures his belief in a postmodern description of modern dance. As a teacher, philosopher, and choreographer, you might say he was very much like John Dewey in terms of valuing aesthetics, all art forms, and experience.

HAWKINS'S THEORY OF DANCE, EXPERIENCE, AND ART

My life's experience is made of the way I controlled my negativity twenty-four hours a day. My relations with my students are the consequences purely of the patterns of my thought in the way I believe in growth, healthy-mindedness, harmony, health, and love. (1992, p. 71)

This statement by Hawkins provides the frame for understanding how dance as art and experience came to be the core of Hawkins's beliefs and actions. From the outside looking in, Hawkins's theory of dance was one of free movement, asymmetry, exploration of any part of the body as storyteller, and feeling life. Each and every movement of dance conveyed some idea of human experience. Hawkins once stated that "the most beautiful thing, the most exciting thing about modern dance is that nobody can define it." Hawkins added, "I conceive of modern dance as a **direction of the human spirit** here in America in the making of art which cannot repeat, relive, rewarm, standstill, copy or revert or keep corpses alive" (1992, p. 89).

When Hawkins spoke of this idea, obviously many agreed that modern dance was not ballet. At the time, that was about all that could be agreed on. This was a period of tremendous development and change in the history of dance globally and in the history of Western modern dance in particular. Modern dance was evolutionary and, as in Hawkins's technique, was idiosyncratic; techniques were named for the teachers and their schools, such as the Martha Graham, Merce Cunningham, Erick Hawkins, and Twyla Tharp techniques. In addition, international choreographers such as Maurice Béjart made regular teaching residencies and performed regularly in New York City. In fact, New York was home to multiple international companies on a regular basis for short and long periods of time. This practice continues today. For example, although in reading any current issue of *Dance Magazine*, you will find features on dance around the world as a global village, nearly every major dance company worldwide still makes it a goal to perform in New York City. Along with its already existing ballet centers, this new movement made New York City a center of the Western dance world, which allowed it to feature the innovative, the unusual, and the provocative movements in dance history, a situation that continues to the present day. Virtually every existing Western modern dance company evolved from the work of the preceding pioneers. Still others developed techniques in other countries, but they eventually came to New York— for example, the great experimentalists Hanya Holm and Mary Wigman. Many hybrids emerged that mixed ballet and modern dance. More intriguing, they originated their studios in New York and then relocated to other cities to continue the development and evolution of modern dance. One example is the Robert Joffrey Ballet Company, which now calls Chicago its home, thus broadening the geographic locations for dance as experience in the Western view of modern dance. Historically, Hawkins's ideas were needed to shape new interpretations of long-held notions of dance. He focused on the intensity of experience as the basis for the creation of any given dance. He stressed the need for freedom of movement and expression. He always worked in collaboration with musicians, composers, dancers, and other artists.

Dewey, Hawkins, and Paulo Freire inspired me as a qualitative researcher and oral historian. Freire, as the creator of critical pedagogy, urges that we work toward a critical enlightenment and thus emancipation. He modeled for us in education and other disciplines the critique of economic determinism and the importance of art and of desire and forced us to see the wisdom of critical thought and action. He reminds me of Hawkins and Dewey in this way, for they also wished to spend their energy on living life and representing it in the art form of dance or poetry or narrative writing to build up a history of stories. They were not interested in tearing down other cultural workers or philosophers. As a result, it was a natural progression for me as an educator and researcher to gravitate to oral history. I see oral history as an orientation that can help my students come to their own emancipation. It is the reason I like to showcase their work in the examples in this book. Each one validates the who, what, why, and where of research as an art and as lived experience. In that vein, let us turn to a good example of the work of John E. Hawkins, who interviewed Lacy Lane, a well-known arts educator. Here John uses his oral history interviews from our class to come up with initial themes that inspire him to go forward along these lines for his dissertation.

CASE IV.1.
ca~

Equity and Access: Art Thou in the Arts?

BY JOHN E. HAWKINS

INTERVIEW INTRODUCTION

Ms. Lacy Lane was selected for the interview project. She is well versed in the academic nature of the arts and can clearly articulate the impact of current accountability reform on making the arts accessible to all students. Her current employment allows her to serve over 150 schools in the capacity of Senior Coordinator for Visual Arts in Polk County. Professional affiliations include senior advisor for the College Board and president of the Florida Art Educators Association. She is revered by her peers not only because of her formal titles but for her dedicated service to teachers in advancing their artistic instruction.

Two interviews held on February 19 and 23, 2009, revealed a variety of perspectives relative to the importance of arts to our society, the impact of high-stakes testing on the arts in the nation's public schools, and the value of the arts in teaching creativity and problem-solving skills. Both performance exercises of interviewing will be referenced as a pilot study for my dissertation.

I have chosen to study the arts, as the arts have been an all-encompassing element in my life. My artistic journey began in the fourth grade while playing saxophone in the intermediate-grades band and currently surrounds my services as secretary for an international arts organization supporting arts schools: Arts Schools Network. My past experiences serve as stimuli in strengthening my interest in the current state of the arts in public school education.

The question proposed in this research design is, In this age of school reform accountability in Florida, how do we construct a pedagogical framework about the arts and promote their expansion in our high schools? While researching this question, the philosophical assumptions are framed to expose the breadth of the research question. The current state of reality in arts education is that secondary public school students are limited in opportunities to experience the arts. Specifically, mandates associated with accountability reform have minimized flexibility in course availability and selection. It can be found in varying degrees at both the elementary and secondary levels. Lacy Lane abridged this ontology during our second interview.

> But in Florida, Level 1 and Level 2 students (low performers) are routinely denied access to the arts. They don't have room in their schedules for electives and they don't get it. That happens early on. Children are pulled out of elementary school art classes to, uh, go into pullout programs where they are hammered with more stuff, with more stuff that they didn't get very well the first time. And it just, that to me is our biggest issue. And I am all for accountability and I am all for some kind of testing. I think it keeps us honest. But not at the expense of children. And I think that's where we are now. If I had to think that I had to go to middle school and I couldn't enjoy something that at least part of the day, you know me, I'd

just be thinking of a way to get out of there. And wait till I am 16. I can guarantee you I am out of there. And that's what we've done. And I truly believe that every child has got to learn to read and write. I, I think that we do ourselves a disservice socially, society, if we don't teach children. But I also think that we have to be able to give them something that they love; that they enjoy doing.

Ms. Lane echoed my sentiments on the arts:

To me, the arts . . . and it's not just the visual arts, but all of the arts. First of all, they're our history, they're our culture. They help to define who we are. And I think it's so important that our students touch that. And you know what I used to tell my kids? You're not gonna be a Michelangelo and you're not gonna be Leonardo. And that's okay. But [what] I really want you to do is to be a great taxpayer, who values public art. I want you to be the person who knows the difference between hotel art and art that you want in your home, and art that you want in public places. So, if you take that away from what we do here [pause], you've taken so much. The other thing that I think the arts help students do [sigh] and again, we talked about it a few minutes ago. They empower kids. [pause] I think about the number of students I've worked with through the years in visual arts and for one reason or another had learning disabilities, had, had families who really didn't give a flyin' flip about what happened to their kids. You know? And that I saw, it doesn't mean their parents don't care.

Secondly, I am a White middle-class male attempting to transcend middle-class values as viewed through the window of White privilege. McLaren and Kincheloe (2007) describe privileged people as justifying their privilege "by internalizing the myth that hard work, fair assessment, and equal access to institutions of power create equal opportunities for success and failure" (p. 61). Consequently, oppression is the face of the failures of an individual. They also remind us that privileged people typically do not want to create equity if it means losing their privileges, whether it be gender, race, or social class.

Conversely, No Child Left Behind [NCLB] is the catalyst for school reform and supposedly closing achievement gaps between subgroups. High-stakes testing has become an obsession at both the state and federal levels. Former Florida Governor Jeb Bush serves as only one example of the opposite position in devaluing arts instruction in public schools as evidence of his proposal to discontinue the mandatory fine arts credit. Additionally, artists are in a tug-of-war over classic arts versus pop arts. Curricular wars in the arts are also abundant. Thus the use of personal, narrative research will support my ability to describe this situation.

Ms. Lane encapsulated the current state of policy as lived out in some districts in the state of Florida:

> I am hearing from other districts that they are cutting art teachers and music teachers. Um, I, I really . . . I think high-stakes testing . . . and that's that thing about high-stakes testing. Like, that we use, to me . . . again I go back to thinking and we have to teach these kids how to think. And sometimes I don't think that the high-stakes testing . . . all that prep for that . . . does not do that. Um, the other thing that I think is really, really sad is if you're a Level 1 student or a Level 2 student within this particular school district, and I think that is true for all others in this state, most of the time you do not have an elective, so you're denied, not only do you have trouble because you can't read or do math but you're also denied the ability to be a part of something that for one reason or another you might be really good at. And feel . . . I have kids that learn to read because they were in an arts class. I've seen that. Sitting them in these prep classes doing the same thing over and over again isn't going to teach them to read. So . . . I do think it is going to have a big impact on us before it is over. I don't exactly know how much. But if things continue as they are in education in Florida, it is going to take our system 20 years to recover from what is happening to it right now. I really believe that. And, you know, when I started teaching in this district we may have had 30 art teachers . . . visual arts, and I've watched that grow, and grow, and grow. We now have an art teacher in every elementary school. We have an art teacher in all of the middle schools and high schools. [Sigh] And it just breaks my heart to see that taken away. If that happens. You know, I've heard our superintendent say, "I'm holding on." Well, you were there in the same meeting. "If I can, to art and music teachers." Don't know. It's sad.

Each of my interviews with four arts educators will be detailed individually and themes will be extrapolated.

THEMES, CATEGORIES, AND SUBTHEMES FOUND IN THE PERFORMANCE EXERCISE INTERVIEWS

Two culminating themes surfaced during the two interviews. They are **arts and culture** and **arts in education**. Within those themes there are numerous categories and subthemes. Some of the subthemes are contained in multiple categories.

The **first category is that of public perception of the arts** and can be found in both themes. It is also inclusive of the five subthemes: understanding, diversity, academic nature of the arts, design in society, and a belief that the arts are nonacademic.

Ms. Lane revealed her personal passion when our conversations gravitated towards the enrollment of students of color in the arts, as well as the perceived level of understanding of the arts by parents of students of color.

Addressing the category of public perception in the arts, Ms. Lane continually spoke of the importance of the subtheme **design in society**. Clothing and malls serve as only two easy examples of design infiltrating every facet of our life. There was a point in time where the arts were considered unnecessary and simply "fluff." Yet, attitudes have shifted towards parents valuing the arts as part of their children's lives. She connects her views on design to diversity via recent arts events that she has attended. Through those functions, she paints a picture of vast scale of students and parents. Referring to the diverse attendance at the opening of a recent visual arts exhibit at the Polk Museum of Art, she said:

> It was pretty powerful to look out and see all the different kinds of parents. Tattoos, baseball caps, you know, whatever. But they were there because they recognize there is some power in what's going on here and they want their children to have that experience. They may not understand it. You know, I really relate to that. It is so much like my folks. They didn't understand it. They didn't understand it, but they wanted me to have it.

Diversity is a topic embedded throughout much of the interviews. Yet probably the most vivid example of diversity is her example of Shepherd Fairey. Fairey is a former skateboard and street artist who now has designed a clothing line called Tag. He also designed the iconic poster of Barack Obama:

> Well, I am thinking about tagging and Shepherd Fairey, but you, certainly he is not a subgroup. But that is where he started. And, and I think about some of the other people who are up and coming, and maybe their aesthetic and my aesthetic didn't start in the same place, but somewhere along the line, and maybe because of Advanced Placement and everything I've done there, I don't know. But, it's like, I appreciate it. And I don't think

it matters where you start. I mean, if it's a eh, eh, world music class or if it's a hip hop music class, or if it's whatever. You've got to hook 'em. And if you can touch them, if you can get them interested, the rest of the stuff comes. Because if they're interested in that, here's history. Here's all this art history that comes and you start wanting to know more, and more, and more. And you have to learn about that because you want to know more about how you can be better at what you do. I don't think it matters where you start. I think it just matters that you've got to start.

The **second category, creativity, includes the subthemes of creativity versus compliance, process and problem solving, and teacher-directed work under the theme of arts in education.** It also has connectivity to the theme of arts and culture via the subtheme, once again, of a design society. In our second interview, Ms. Lane said the following regarding the heightened awareness of design in our society:

> I think Pink (2006) probably said it best. We've moved beyond function. You know, now it is about form. How it looks. And is it aesthetically pleasing, and who is in a better place to do that than visual artists? And I think it's all about creativity now. I don't care what field you're in. Um, it's about being able to think and, of course, my favorite term, solve problems. And, and that's where I see the arts.

Following this conversation, Ms. Lane brilliantly merged the creativity, problem solving, and design in a few simple statements:

> You know. Who's going to solve that issue of power? You know. It's going to be some little guy, sitting somewhere, who has been taught to think outside the box. And I think that's what the visual arts do. We teach kids to think outside the page. And you know, he, he [Pink] makes all sorts of statements about people who are hiring now want to look at artist portfolios, and one of the most interesting things I remember is talking to the architect who did all of this one day here at the school. He and I were just sitting there, it was at a meeting.

Creativity versus compliance and process versus problem solving were selected due to the place of prominence the arts hold in the 21st century and the arts serving as conduit in transmitting problem-solving skills (Pink, 2006). Compliance was judged against creativity due to Ms. Lane's extensive explanation on creative art versus teacher-directed art. For example, she said problem solving is paralyzing for some students. Elaborating further, she said:

> In education, we're really good at telling students to regurgitate. The key to success is, tell them what they [teachers] want to hear. And so you move into an art class, and some of these kids are really, really uncomfortable because it's the first time in their educational career that someone has not told them what's right. You know, some of the hardest kids I've ever had to work with are my very, very, what I put in quotation marks, "good students."

The continual creative process, in which students are immersed in quality arts instruction, is what promotes transcendent thinking.

Thirdly, **the category arts for society** embraces the concept of White privilege in both themes. The subtheme [of] equity and access to the arts is found under the theme arts in education, and the long-lasting effects of inequity and limited access produce the subtheme [of] social stratification under arts and culture. When sharing her thoughts on White privilege, Ms. Lane said:

> I do think that there is some degree of White privilege in what goes on. I mean, just look at our school system. Look. Go over to Eastside. Go to school over there. You know. And I am not saying they don't do a good job, because they do. But, they also deal with a turnover in terms of teachers and half of their kids come to school not speaking English. It's a tremendous turnaround, or turnover in teachers there, or has been traditionally. I think she's [the principal] finally put a stop to that. But, I do think there is some of that. When you go [long pause] when on a Saturday going to the museum is a way of life for you with your child, or reading a book, or whatever. Yeah, I think there is a difference for some parents where survival is going to, to work on Saturday. And getting with your child to read a book is something that you do at the end of the day. It's tough. You're worn out. And I think as middle-class teachers, and I hear this, and, and this is very anecdotal, I mean, you know, this is just how I feel. But I sit in the, the rooms with teachers and I listen to teachers fuss about parents who don't care. Parents who don't care. The majority of us grew up with parents who did care in some way, shape, or form. And I really believe we have parents who care. We do. Circumstance, time, money, prevent them from being in the schools. The bureaucracy of trying to reach someone in the school is enough to drive you crazy [long pause]. Try filling out financial aid papers. I have two degrees. Two graduate degrees, and I throw my

hands up. Now you tell me we want to make it easy for parents. Try to call Lakeland High School and see if you can get through.

Next, Ms. Lane put an exclamation point on her stance regarding White privilege. She was quite vocal about teachers complaining about parents who don't care about their child's education. In fact, she said, "It makes me crazy." With added emphasis on her point that parents actually do care, she said:

> I'll never forget what fellow art educator, Clint Wright, said to me one day and he said it all over this town. He goes, "Patricia." I said, "Yes, Clint." He goes, "They don't keep the best ones at home. They send us the best they've got." And they want the best for them.

The next single category appearing under the theme of arts in education is **literacy in the arts**. This category is an umbrella for the sub-themes of high-stakes testing, achievement, construct, and transfer of processes. This broad category was chosen because it is the center of a web that demonstrates that rigor of quality arts instruction.

Speaking on transference of processes of the arts to general academia, Ms. Lane discussed the arts in relation to mathematics and how mathematicians are required to look at numbers in new ways. In addition, she emphasized the importance of the arts "serving students well in writing and the ability to synthesize new information." However, the most emotional aspect of the interview came when sharing her views on high-stakes testing. Going into immense detail, she spoke of how tracking and ability grouping had imprinted negative lifelong memories in the mind of one of her children. When asked about pullout programs, she spoke of how high-stakes testing is forcing some principals to suspend instruction in the arts:

> You go to any school in this district [Polk County]. It depends upon the principal. It depends on what results the principal is seeing with what they've tried to do. And I can think of one right now where she has no problem pulling students out of art over and over and over again. Because she has seen a rise in her reading scores. And she needed to see a rise in her scores. We'll never get kids back in a program there that will work, um, until she's gone. Because it has worked for her. You know and what, what a lot of principals don't understand is there are ways to do it. There are other schools who do great things that don't do pullouts. And I don't

have a problem with pullout, if you're going to pull kids out, let's do it equitably. You know. You take them from art once, you take them from music once, you take them from PE [physical education] once.

Next is the category of **accountability reform**, which also meshes with both themes. Subthemes include Florida's implementation of NCLB, core versus noncore courses, and how legislators make decisions pertaining to the arts. Regarding decisions that are made at the legislative level, Ms. Lane stated:

I really believe, and five years ago I would not have said this, but I really believe there is a concerted effort, in this country, by certain people, to separate and deny classes of people. Access to quality education. And sometimes when I say that and I really articulate that, I think oh, my goodness. I sound like one of those conspiracy theorists. But I really do believe that's true. I think, proven right now by what we are facing in Florida, we have legislators whose children are not in public schools. They're not funding what we need to have funded in order to provide an education for students. If we have quality education, people will want the fine arts in their children's lives. Parents [pause] parents know and can see when kids do well. And you know what? They usually do well when they get involved in some aspect of the arts because it gives them, that, that ability to make judgments about themselves. To, you know, and I hate to use the term *better*, but to become better people, better students. Just higher achievers.

Elaborating further, she spoke of the collective voice that educators have, yet teachers are not known for their voting prowess. With heightened voice conveying her passion, she spoke of her own advocacy in encouraging educators to vote and furthering the cause of arts education. She supported her claims as she humorously shared [a story] about her letters to legislators:

I am writing letters to my legislators. I am probably on a list somewhere that says, "Watch out for this woman." But that's okay. You know, I think if we're not vocal, if we don't say what we need to say then . . . they just continue to do what they do. You know, politician J. D. Alexander spent a million dollars to be elected to the position he holds now. A million dollars [repeated slowly for emphasis]. And you know, he's got a lot more than that. So, the next election that he decides to embrace, I am sure he's going after the federal position when that becomes open. Um, and he'll get that. I mean, he really will. I don't want him representing me. First of all, he doesn't know how I live. And what is important to him [pause] does not take into account our students who need him the most. He doesn't understand.

Finally, we reach the last category, which is **professional development**. The subthemes include teacher training in the arts and reading, as well as suspended subjectivity. Suspended subjectivity is important because it discounts the belief that the arts are subjects without criteria and are merely left to individual preferences. In our second interview, Ms. Lane was asked to describe the qualitative grading of advanced-placement art as compared to another subject in general academia. Her response immediately addressed the concept of subjectivity:

> The thing I know with the arts, everyone believes that they are so subjective. And, you know that, therefore grading has to be subjective with it, and that is just not so. I mean, there are rubrics that we follow in the AP studio art course that are based on sound usage of the principles of design and composition. Now, I think the thing that makes this so important, that we are able to train people, and we spend lots of time up front training each one of the readers so that they are able to put away, to put away their personal biases and adhere to the rubric. Now, when we train people, when we speak with them, one of the examples I always use is, I love red. Red is the color choice in my life. And I also love pattern. So if you really want to sucker me into something, paint it red and put a little pattern and throw a little glitz, because I also like sequins a lot. And if you do that, when I first look at it, I am going to go, "Wow!" But if then I take my rubric and I use that rubric to determine whether or not this piece fulfills each one of those standards, if it doesn't, . . . although I still like that red and I still like that pattern, and the sequins make me giggle, I know that it hasn't met the standard. And it's that training with each one of the readers, the potential readers, that I think makes all of the difference in the world. We first have to come to a common agreement about what is composition.

Teacher training can be seen in the example of advanced-placement courses through the College Board above, as well as Ms. Lane's commitment to teacher training within the school district. Additional training can be seen through her role as president of the Florida Art Education Association.

> One of the questions that I ask teachers a lot as I go out and see them is "If you were asked to do this, would you be bored? And if you're bored, why on earth do you believe that your students aren't?" I believe that when we teach we have to set up problems for students to solve. We have to teach them how to think. And you do that in the visual arts so easily. You don't do it if all you are about is teaching process. And process is wonderful, but you have to give them something else. I offer them lots of professional development for teachers that I serve now. . . . I have workshops. I have professional learning communities. I offer, I have training for new teachers. Just to help them with all those issues that trip up beginning teachers. . . . There is just so much that they don't understand. Behavior is always an issue with most beginning teachers. Behavior management, classroom management. And having a safe place that they can talk about those problems I think is a real help to them.

This concept paper has described how two interviews helped me find a design for my dissertation. The dissertation will identify themes through what Creswell (2007) calls a "within-case analysis" (p. 75). Themes will also be extrapolated across all four cases of four arts educators.

∽

In this example, the researcher finds social justice issues embedded in his major themes and in his categories of analysis. This will later be useful for his interpretation of the data. He is in the initial stages of using guidelines that many may use in the research process. As he looks at the data after transcribing the interviews, he begins his data analysis by doing the following:

1. Looking for statements in the data that lead to empirical assumptions.
2. Using narrative vignettes extracted from the interview transcripts.
3. Scanning any documents provided by the narrator.
4. Including interpretive commentary.

5. Including or beginning a theoretical discussion from the data.

6. Describing the role of the researcher.

7. Describing ethical issues brought up in the data.

Thus the process of analysis is in play. John has also taken photographs of Lacy and will most likely use them at some point. Thus he is expanding his range of evidence with photographic media and will use his judgment to select which photographs are appropriate in the final version of this study. In addition to the preceding list, I add the following, which I ask my students to do in their work:

1. Identify any points of serendipity that occur in the data.

2. Develop a metaphor to capture your findings.

3. Describe your own creativity.

4. Look for what doesn't fit in the study or statements of the narrator.

5. Look for contradictions and identify and explain them to the best of your ability.

These, of course, are only some guidelines for teaching the critical approach to looking at data. All are designed to capture a story of someone's lived experience. Here as well, the social justice issue of access to the arts for some but not all high school students will be an area for research in the future. In addition, throughout this book, the various examples indicate the individual styles people have of using direct sections of the interview transcript and their own styles of narrative writing. All the examples presented in this text also point to the need for and importance of reflecting on the role of the researcher. Researchers in this genre need to be able to reflect on what they have done. Consider this next example, by Kay M. Wigman. It is her reflection on returning from three observations at a knitting store called Knit 'n Knibble in Tampa, Florida. This example includes her beginning observations and descriptions excerpted from the entire work.

CASE IV.2.

༄

Introductory Remarks to the Observation Assignment, Followed by Observation 3 at the Site and Reflections on the Role of the Researcher

BY KAY M. WIGMAN

We don't see things as they are, we see things as we are.
—ANAIS NIN

Knit 'n Knibble is located on the west side of South Dale Mabry Highway, a major thoroughfare lined with businesses and restaurants that passes through many neighborhoods in the city of Tampa. The store lies on the eastern edge of the Palma Ceia West, a neighborhood within the city limits of Tampa, Florida. The neighborhood is a part of the South Tampa District, where urban revitalization has produced an area where businesses and neighborhoods mingle together. The bordering neighborhoods to the east included Palma Ceia and Gulfview. This area has been home to Tampa residents since the early 1920s. The neighborhoods have a wide range of home styles lining the red brick roads that are shaded by enormous live oak trees. These houses are nestled back from the hustle and bustle of the main roads.

West Palma Ceia is a neighborhood encompassing portions of two zip codes: 33609 and 33629. The geographic boundaries of Palma Ceia are San Obispo to the south, Morrison Avenue to the north, Dale Mabry Highway to the east, and Lois Avenue to the west (a recent report of City of Tampa Neighborhood and Community Relations). . . . As of the 2000 census the neighborhood had a population of 2,531 residing in 1,127 households.

I selected Knit 'n Knibble for a nonparticipant observational study because it is a unique store in the Greater Tampa Bay area that attracts individuals from across the state for the purpose of knitting and crocheting. While there are other major chain stores, such as Jo-Ann Fabrics and Michael's Crafts for the purchasing of yarn and accessories, Knit 'n Knibble is one of only five shops dedicated to yarn art in the Greater Tampa Bay Area. It is the only store located in Tampa (the other stores are located in Palm Harbor, Seminole, and St. Petersburg, Florida). I am familiar with this location due to my interest in knitting and crochet as hobbies. I was introduced to crochet by my grandmother when I was

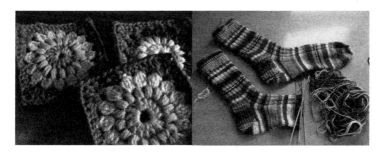

*Crochet granny squares recently made into a dog blanket, and a pair of knit
socks currently still on my knitting needles.*

a young girl. By age 8, I could crochet granny squares and sew them
together to make an afghan. In 2005 I was introduced to knitting by
Polly, the teacher from the classroom next door to my classroom. As
my interest in knitting grew, I wanted to take classes and find a wider
variety of yarns. Knit 'n Knibble became my source for both knitting
instruction and high-quality supplies such as silk and cashmere yarns.
I am a frequent visitor to this location.

On any given visit to Knit 'n Knibble, I would encounter individuals
from all walks of life—business executives, teachers, students, stay-at-
home moms, young children, and retirees. Both men and women alike
would be in the store, although the clientele is predominately female
knitters. The majority of visitors to Knit 'n Knibble are regular customers. Some are from the local city of Tampa, but others travel from as far
away as Orlando and Jacksonville. It is the nature of this small shop
to pull together people across the boundaries of age, race, gender, and
economic groups for a common hobby that drew me to this location for
my nonparticipant observational study. I knew there would be much to
observe and write about in this eclectic setting.

Note: Kay observed three times. Here is her third observation, followed by a reflection on her role as a researcher.

OBSERVATION 3: ONE KNITTER'S REFUGE

After my first two visits to observe Knit 'n Knibble, a major theme
became apparent among the visitors to this shop. I noticed that the

majority of visitors to the knit shop came here to relax, socialize, and escape the pressures of their everyday lives. This was evidenced by comments such as: "I just need to knit something!" "Knitting calms me down," "Finally, I can escape for a little bit," "I love the process, the sense of accomplishment, I have to have something in my hands, it calms me down," and "After 33 years my husband is finally getting it. The more time I spend here, the less time I spend yelling at him, or spending money on stupid things!" It is as though Knit 'n Knibble is a refuge for these individuals.

With this theme in mind, I selected Polly as the individual knitter that I would observe. This choice was purposeful in that I have a personal relationship with Polly and am aware of the undue amount of stress she currently has in her life. Currently, Polly is a full-time reading teacher at an urban high school in South Tampa. Her husband recently underwent emergency surgery for bleeding on the brain. Events surrounding this surgery became more stressful when the drill used to create burr holes in his skull failed after he was under anesthesia but before surgery commenced. Her husband had to be transferred to a different hospital in an unfamiliar part of town for Polly. Adding to Polly's anxieties was the fact that her 3-year-old Lhasa apso dog, Duchess, is suffering from renal failure and requires regular injections of fluid and medications.

Polly and I often go together to Knit 'n Knibble either after a full day of work or on a Saturday. When I began my observations, Polly had taken a 1½-week leave of absence from work in order to be with her husband during his surgery and recovery. My final observation was on Saturday, January 17th, 2009, from 12:00 P.M. to 1:00 P.M. Polly and I were spending the day together attending to things she needed to get done, including some shopping and visiting with her husband in the rehabilitation facility, where he had been transferred to for recovery. Our trip to Knit 'n Knibble this day was prior to our visit with her husband. Because of our friendship, Polly was aware of my observational project and some of its specific requirements; however, she was unaware of the fact that I had selected her as a specific individual to observe as a part of this project.

Polly was wearing a black-colored suit jacket over a black tank top, with a black skirt patterned with leaves. She was wearing a new pair of earrings given to her by her husband for Christmas. The earrings are square drop earrings set in white gold. Each earring has a center of four blue sapphires surrounded by white diamonds. The drop extension is also lined with white diamonds. On the ring finger of her left hand is a gold ring set with diamonds and dark blue sapphires. She also has a silver watch with gold trim on her left wrist. Also adorning her left wrist is a gold bracelet set with diamonds and blue sapphires.

She sits at the large wooden table in the middle of the knit shop in the chair closest to the doorway to the classroom. I am sitting at the end of the table closest to the cash register. Many of the same knitters from previous observations sit around the table. Kate is sitting across from Polly and continues to work on the brown-flecked sweater. Another knitter, whom we do not know, is sitting next to Polly beginning a red lacy shawl.

Kate inquires, "How is your husband doing?"

Polly responds pleasantly, "He is in rehab now and is doing well, thank you for asking."

Kate continues, "So his brain surgery went okay?"

"Yes, but the brain drill didn't work, so they had to take him all the way to [another] hospital on the other end of town to actually do the

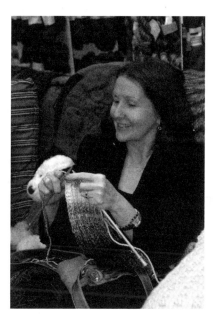

Polly smiling and knitting a scarf.

surgery!" Polly answers. "This hat is for him, since he had to have all of his hair shaved off for the surgery."

Polly is knitting a striped hat on silver circular knitting needles. It has a double-rolled edge in cranberry. The first roll was created by knitting in stockinette stitch (when you alternate a knit row with a purl row), and the second roll is created by reversing the pattern. Stockinette stitch creates a smooth side and a bumpy side to the fabric. The hat has a total of three cranberry stripes, alternating with a multicolor yarn consisting of navy blue, heather green, and cranberry as the main yarn. The smooth side of the yarn was always the multicolored yarn, and the bumpy side of the hat was the cranberry-colored yarn.

Polly further explains, "I've knit him a hat for every day of the week. So far he has a yellow one, a red one, this one, and a brown one. The nurses all comment on his hats. I've even had one nurse ask if I would knit her a hat. So I showed her all the hats I had brought back after washing them and let her pick one."

Polly continues to knit the hat. She switches from the silver circular needle to four bamboo double-pointed needles of the same diameter. "I've finally learned how to do this part, the double points, I used to just make Kay do it for me, but she finally made me learn how to do it myself." She smiles and laughs. "It's a good thing, too, I don't think Kay would want to do the finish work on as many hats as I've made the past week!"

One of the women asks Polly, "Do you get to knit while you are visiting with him?"

Polly responds, "It's about all I do, because he is usually sleeping. He calls me after I go home and is mad at me because he doesn't remember that I was there. I tell him to look around the room at the pictures, his clothes put away, and the other decorations, and I ask him who he thinks put all those things there. So I knit! What else is there to do?"

Then she laughs. "The next hat is for me! I'm doing it in this black and white marbled yarn. Then I'm going to make a matching scarf. I better not let him see it or he will want this one, too," she jokes.

The women around the table offer her encouragement and share stories of hospital stays. One woman shares a story of her last hospital visit. A male staffer shares a story of when his mom was last in the hospital. And others share stories of stays their relatives had in hospitals.

Polly says she wishes he would hurry up and come home. Others joke about husbands—how they take their "good old time" no matter what they do.

With this, Polly shares how much her life has changed since her husband became ill. One year ago he suffered a stroke. The stroke left him with left-side impairments and swallowing issues. She has had to blend his food up like baby food for the past year. Recently he had a feeding tube placed because he had lost nearly forty pounds. But at least he had been home for the past year and was able to keep her company. Now she says, "This is a big change in my life . . . being all by myself, cleaning and cooking. I don't really care for it. But I know that I have to get used to it; there is the chance that he may never come home. He may have to go to a nursing home if he needs 'round the clock care because I have to go back to work. Actually, I start back on Monday!"

Again, the women and one man in the shop offer encouragement to Polly.

Polly transfers the attention to the knitter beside her at the table by asking what she is making. This woman shares that she is making a lacy shawl, but she is having difficulty because the needles are slippery and shiny, making it difficult to see her yarn. Polly asks her what type of needles she is knitting with. The woman responds that they are Addi needles (known to be some of the best needles in knitting circles). Polly says that she has never seen Addi needles that look like that and wants to know what type they are. This set of needles has a red cable joining the two metal needles. Most Addi Turbo needles have a silver cable joining the needles. A different woman at the table responds that those are needles specifically made for lace. The red cable makes it easier to see as you knit the intricate lace patterns. Polly jokes, "I want all of my needles to have that red cable so I can see better on all of my knitting."

Caroline, Knit 'n Knibble's owner, comes over to the table at this point and hears Polly's comment. She tells Polly that she can have almost all of her needles in this style. Caroline explains that they also have the added benefit of having very tapered tips for precise knitting and the needles are brass; but the smallest length they come in are 24 inches, so they won't work for Polly's hats. Polly jokes, "Well, then, they should make a pair just for me and my hats."

Caroline asks Polly how her husband is doing, and Polly gives her a condensed version of the update she had been giving to everyone at the table.

Polly changes the subject to the purple snood (a long knit hat that looks similar to a hair net) that Jenna is wearing. "I want to make one of these for my student assistant . . . not that I don't already have enough projects started." Caroline calls Jenna over to assist Polly in finding the pattern and yarn. Jenna tells Polly that the pattern is free, but it is found on a website called *Ravelry.com*. This website is a social networking website that you must join. Jenna tells Polly that it usually takes a couple of days to get an invite to the network once you e-mail a request. Polly proudly tells Jenna that she is already a member.

Jenna goes over to the computer beside the knitting table and pulls up the website. Polly gets up from the table so Jenna can show her how to find the pattern and download it. Polly is comfortable with the pattern and wants to look at yarn. At this time, another woman asks if anyone is sitting in the chair that Polly has been sitting in. Polly calls back, "I was, but I'll move my stuff, I'm looking at yarn and will sit on the sofas when I'm done." She picks up her knitting and places it back in her black and silver bag. She then picks up her purse and her knitting bag and places [them] on the denim sofa closest to the table. Once done, she returns to Jenna and the wall of yarn across from the cash register. She and Jenna have a discussion about which yarns will work best for

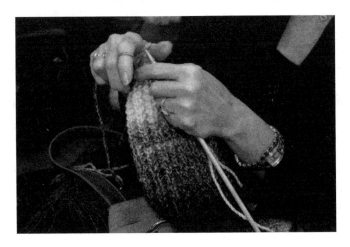

Polly's scarf, which she is knitting for herself, grows in length.

the snood. Jenna recommends cotton so the snood will not be so hot in Florida weather, but to be careful [so] that the cotton will retain some stretch and bounce back to shape, since it needs to sit snug on the head. Many types of cotton will stretch with time and not recover their original shape.

Polly decides she needs to ask her student assistant what color she will want before buying the yarn. With that, she goes to the denim sofa and picks up her black and white yarn to begin working on the scarf she mentioned previously. As she knits the scarf, she updates others on the status of her husband. She is talking, sipping on her tea, knitting, laughing, and generally relaxing until she notices that I have stepped away from the knitting table and put my notebook away.

"You're done with your project?" she inquires with a bit of trepidation.

"I'm done with today's observation," I reply.

"Are you going to knit?" she pleads.

"I'll knit if you want to stay longer."

"Yes, sit down and knit. I'm not ready to go back out there just yet. I want to escape for just a little bit longer. And I want to see you knit on that purple sock of yours. Then we will go visit."

So I sit on the denim sofa across from Polly, the same spot where I began my observations on January 7, 2009, and pull out my purple Celtic braid sock and begin knitting in the round, expanding the insole of the sock. At that point Polly asks me who I had decided to do my observation on. I tell Polly that it is her. She says, "Well, I'm honored and I hope I gave you enough to write about. Gosh, I think I kept talking about the same thing, my husband!"

REFLECTION ON MY ROLE AS AN OBSERVER

Given the opportunity and all the time in the world, I would conduct this study as a fully immersed participant and conduct a narrative study (Creswell, 2007, pp. 53–55). I found that my position within this community gave me an "insider's view" and at times prevented me from being a nonparticipant. And many times, I found myself frustrated not being able to interact with the individuals around me. I wanted to talk with them, ask questions, and conduct informal interviews to gain more access into the culture of the Knit 'n Knibble.

With this additional time, I would focus on a few things that I noticed as a result of my three observations. First, I would want to observe the difference between a clinic and a class. In both cases instruction is being given, but the clinic is free. This comparison would provide some interesting insight by observing how the staff interacts with the knitters. Is there a difference? How do the knitters behave during these two different sessions? Next, I would want to spend time observing the interactions between the regular knitters and new customers to the shop. Are these sets of individuals treated differently by the staff? How does an individual feel as they enter a shop that is full of regular knitters engaged in social activities? How does a knitter new to the shop become a regular knitter accepted by the rest of the regular knitters? Finally, I would want to conduct interviews. I would want to question different knitters about why they come to this shop. What does the shop mean to them?

Given more time, another approach I could employ would be to conduct a multiple case study. As I mentioned earlier, there are a total of five shops dedicated to yarn art in the Greater Tampa Bay area. I would use the same observational procedures at one or more of the other shops and do a comparison case study looking for similar themes to emerge from the data (Creswell, 2007).

SELF-EVALUATION

As a scientist I have been trained to observe physical and natural events and occurrences and record them in detail. When asked to make observations, I find myself reaching for my ruler to be precise and accurate in my measurements. I want to measure, measure, measure, photograph, photograph, and photograph. I fill pages upon pages of quad-ruled composition notebooks with field notes while studying sponges or other invertebrates in their natural habitat. When I conduct experiments, I painstakingly record every variable I manipulate, every procedure I carry out, and the exact measured results. I then write the laboratory reports in the dry, lifeless, passive voice I have been trained to use in scientific writing. While I love science, experimentation, and field work, and the accuracy required to conduct and convey my finding, I have always found the writing to be a laborious task.

This task was different and challenging for me in several ways. First, instead of focusing in on one tiny small chemical molecule and its reactions inside of an organism (small scale), I was observing numerous organisms (humans) in a niche within their environment (large scale). Capturing the essence of everything, physical setting and activity, was a daunting task. The second challenge for me was finding a way to focus on pockets of action. I had considered Knit 'n Knibble to be a small location to observe. The preconceived notion had me trying to record all of the action within the shop at a single sitting. I came to realize that there are smaller pockets of activity within the shop. For example, the main knitting table, each classroom, the sofa setting, and even the area around the cash register are all individual areas that would warrant focused observation. Each area would provide a different perspective of the shop. The final challenge for me was to convert my visual memory into written word. I know that my memory records images in the form of pictures and movies. I can usually describe these movies in a stream-of-consciousness fashion, but putting the "mind-images" into written word was difficult. I especially found it difficult to find a note-taking style to invoke these images at a later time. During each observation I attempted to write detail-filled notes. In doing so, I felt as though I was missing the action or that the images in my mind were fragmented. For future observations, I will use an unobtrusive video camera to record what I am observing as a way of checking my notes.

Despite having a plan of action prior to my arrival, I found myself having difficulty focusing on one task. My plan was to conduct three observations, each at a different time, with a different focus (setting, action, one individual). Although I had visited this location many times and felt I knew the setting, once I focused on describing the physical setting I became overwhelmed by the sheer amount of things to be described. I began by sitting down and looking around, trying to decide a logical order to begin describing the setting. I began writing, and writing, and writing. As I looked at my watch I realized that time was moving by faster than I anticipated and I was not capturing as many details as necessary. I had the forethought to take my camera with me and decided that I needed to begin taking photographs. Originally, I had planned to snap a few photos to check my written description against, but as my first hour of observation drew to an end, I found myself taking as many photos as possible. I realized I simply could not capture the tremendous amounts of objects that created the setting. In fact, my use of photography was almost a knee-jerk reaction to avoid falling short on this part of the assignment. As it turns out, this knee-jerk reaction is a natural tendency toward building my own compendium of data collection approaches (Creswell, 2007) for my qualitative research.

Reviewing what I have written, I realize that in some cases, I may have added unnecessary detail. I have read several books set within knit shops, such as *Family Tree* by Barbara Delinsky and *Twenty Wishes* by Debbie Macomber. Both of these books evoke images of knit shops similar to Knit 'n Knibble, but their description is mingling with the storyline. Reading my description of Knit 'n Knibble in some cases still reminds me of the mechanical descriptions I would use in my scientific papers, rather than the vivid, lively narration in novels that evoke images in my mind.

To further compound this issue, I found myself getting distracted by things outside of my focus for the visit. I was easily distracted by the action in the shop to the point that I wanted to pick up my own knitting and immerse myself in the atmosphere. This is easily a side effect of my familiarity with the setting and the fact that I was there for a different reason than my normal visits. This tendency was one I had to fight during each visit in an attempt to maintain my nonparticipant status. There were numerous times I was drawn into conversation and broke my role of nonparticipant to find myself in a participatory role, "going native," as Creswell (2007) refers to this phenomenon. It will take more practice to remain in the nonparticipatory role. I look forward to conducting a study where I am not among people I am familiar with so that I practice observing a stranger, as suggested by Janesick (2004) as a stretching exercise. Evaluating the differences in my description of individuals I am familiar with versus someone I am unfamiliar with will make for a revealing self-study.

During my writing I continually referred to my notes and photographs to check my details for accuracy. As I did so, I found I became more comfortable with my descriptive writing. My personal overarching goal with this assignment was to see if the narrative writing style of qualitative writing would feel comfortable for me, someone trained in scientific technical writing. While I think there is plenty of room for my writing to improve, I can hear myself telling a story as I write. I had my husband read passages of my writing to check the accessibility and the compelling nature of the paper. Ordinarily, when my husband reads and edits documents for my research and course work, he comments, "I don't have a clue what I just read, but I corrected your typos." My husband has visited Knit 'n Knibble with me. This time, when he read, he kept nodding his head and saying, "That sounds like your knitting shop." This verified for me a successful first attempt at a qualitative study. I would like to have others read my observational study and check my descriptions against their perceptions of the shop. For instance, I'd like Polly to read my observation of her. Additionally, I would like Caroline to read my description of the shop. Overall, conducting this study has been a positive experience and has verified that I want to pursue this type of study during my proposal and dissertation.

In this case example, observation enabled Kay, and I hope all my students, to become more reflective on the process of doing research in general but narrative research methods in particular. By practicing observation and writing observations and reflections, one can become better prepared to do interviewing. In the field of oral history and when doing any other type of qualitative interviewing, the interviewer is also an observer of the narrator, even while the interview is being taped. I design the exercises to sharpen observation and interview skills to assist learners in the process of learning to do oral history. The exercises are similar to the exercises the dancer uses to warm up and get ready for a performance. The performance in this case is the final narrative to be written.

FINAL REFLECTIONS

To make sense of oral history, choreographing the story we tell as historians and researchers, art, experience, and inquiry, I return historically to the third chapter of *Art as Experience*, which is titled, "Having an Experience." Dewey begins: "Experience occurs continuously because the interaction of live creature and environing condition is involved in the very process of living" (p. 35). And while Dewey speaks about this in theory as a philosopher/writer, Hawkins writes in the here and now of an actual dance in progress. Hawkins wants us to see the body as the perfect instrument of the lived experience:

> Several times so-called critics have judged the dancers of my company as being "too graceful." How can you be too graceful? How can you obey the laws of movement too much? . . . The answer is a kind of feeling introspected in the body and leads one into doing the correct effort for any movement. The kinesiological rule is to just do the movement . . . The tenderness in the mind takes care of the movement in action. (1992, pp. 133–134)

Similarly, Hawkins wrote:

> One of the reasons we are not accustomed as a culture to graceful movement is because we do not treasure it. The saying among the Greeks of the Athenian supremacy was that the body was to be treasured and great sensitivity was used in the observation of movement. They treasured the body by having many statues of deity . . . maybe they understood that the body is a clear place. (1992, p. 134)

So we can learn from these writers as we look ahead to our qualitative oral history research projects. We can see the lessons here.

1. We learn about the critical importance of experience, imagination, and the resulting artifact as layered and connected.

2. We learn about the power and value of the subjective experience in interpretation of art and artifact.

3. We learn that the landscape of feeling and emotions cannot and should not be avoided when expressing art or artifact.

4. For a researcher to "have the experience" of telling someone's story, the researcher must acknowledge the experience component of empathy, understanding, and the story itself.

5. We celebrate narrative storytelling in whatever form it may take.

One of the reasons I do qualitative research and, specifically, narrative research in the form of oral history is that it is many things, including an art. It is through the arts that a larger audience is most likely reached than in any other curricular or cultural arena. The arts can meet the need of nearly every person, no matter who that person is and no matter where that person is in the world, and so there are social justice implications. In fact, the digital revolution we are experiencing is filled with art, dance, music, poetry, collage, and other art forms stored in the largest digital archives of Google and YouTube. Oral history provides us with understanding of the power of experience, art as experience, and artifacts resulting from the experience, all of which transcend the day-to-day moments of life. In fact, storytelling is its own art form. As we tell stories about the lived experience of our narrator, art illuminates that experience. For me, using poetry, photography, and video whenever possible helps to widen the repertoire of techniques for the person who wishes to become an oral historian and document and interpret a story. So it seems to me that we as qualitative social science researchers are now able to make known to the wider audiences what we know and learn through oral history. As we move ahead to carve out niches such as the arts and their place in the inquiry process we are building a consciousness of experience. To conclude, the words of this proverb are most descriptive:

> Those who say it cannot be done, should not interrupt
> The person doing it.
> —ANCIENT CHINESE PROVERB

Selected Electronic Resources
Websites and Listservs for the Oral Historian

Oral History Association
www.oralhistory.org

The Oral History Association (OHA), established in 1966, seeks to bring together all persons interested in oral history as a way of collecting human memories. With an international membership, the OHA serves a broad and diverse audience. Local historians, librarians and archivists, students, journalists, teachers, and academic scholars from many fields have found that the OHA provides both professional guidance and a collegial environment for sharing information. The OHA encourages standards of excellence in the collection, preservation, dissemination, and uses of oral testimony. The OHA has established a set of goals, guidelines, and evaluation standards for oral history interviews. The association also recognizes outstanding achievement in oral history through an awards program.

H-Oralhist
www.h-net.org/~oralhist

H-Oralhist is a member of the H-Net, Humanities and Social Sciences online initiative. H-Oralhist is a network for scholars and professionals active in studies related to oral history. It is affiliated with the Oral History Association. It contains a wealth of information.

Historical Voices
www.historicalvoices.org

The purpose of Historical Voices is to create a significant, fully searchable online database of spoken word collections spanning the 20th century—the first large-scale repository of its kind. Historical Voices will both provide storage for these digital holdings and display public galleries that cover a variety of interests and topics. Check out this site if you wish to store your digital tales.

Flint Sit-Down Strike (an example from Historical Voices)
www.historicalvoices.org/flint

The Flint Sit-Down Strike site provides an introduction to the sit-down strike for those students or members of the general public who are unaware of the history of this momentous event in American history. It provides an immediacy and personal touch to this historical knowledge through the use of digitized audio files, which contain the actual voices of former sit-downers reminiscing about their experiences.

The OYEZ Project
www.oyez.org

The OYEZ Project is a vast multimedia relational database on the U.S. Supreme Court. It contains abstracts for all leading constitutional decisions of the Court, authoritative oral arguments in streamed media format, and a virtual reality tour of the Supreme Court building.

Earliest Voices: A Gallery from the Vincent Voice Library
www.historicalvoices.org/earliest_voices

Earliest Voices: A Gallery from the Vincent Voice Library is a multimedia site presenting some of the most significant voices captured during the first 50 years of sound recording, 1877–1927. This is a good resource for checking information from that period.

History and Politics Out Loud
www.hpol.org

History and Politics Out Loud is a diverse collection of audio materials—speeches and private communications—relating to U.S. history and politics.

Free Speech Movement Digital Archive
bancroft.berkeley.edu/collections/fsm.html

The Free Speech Movement (FSM) Digital Archives document the role of Mario Savio and other participants in the free speech movement (University of California, Berkeley, September–December 1964), as well as its origins in political protest and civil rights movements and its legacy of political activism and educational reform that can be traced throughout the country and the world down to the present. Please consult the FSM-A (Free Speech Movement Archives) for additional information on the history and activities of the FSM.

American Historical Association
www.historians.org

The American Historical Association (AHA) is a nonprofit membership organization founded in 1884 and incorporated by Congress in 1889 for the promotion of historical studies, the collection and preservation of historical documents and artifacts, and the dissemination of historical research. As the largest historical society in the United States, the AHA provides leadership and advocacy for the profession, fights to ensure academic freedom, monitors professional standards, spearheads essential research in the field, and provides resources and services to help its members succeed. The AHA serves more than 14,000 history professionals, representing every historical period and geographical area. AHA members include K–12 teachers, academics at 2- and 4-year colleges and universities, graduate students, historians in museums, historical organizations, libraries and archives, and government and business, as well as independent historians.

Australia's Oral Histories Online
www.nla.gov.au/ohdir

Australia's Oral History Collections: A National Directory allows users to search tens of thousands of hours of oral history recordings that document Australian life, customs, politics, and traditions.

Columbia University Oral History Program
library.truman.edu/microforms/columbia_oral_history

Columbia University has a collection of over 1,000 transcripts of oral histories of key individuals in the arts, aviation finance and business, law, labor, women professionals, politics, and many other fields.

John F. Kennedy Library, Oral History Interviews
www.jfklibrary.org/Historical

This collection has more than 1,100 interviews related to the Kennedy presidency. It is modeled on the Columbia University oral history program.

Hawaiian Oral History Summarized on the Web
www2.soc.hawaii.edu/css/oral_hist

The Center for Oral History of the University of Hawaii at Manoa's Social Science Research Institute has an extensive, illustrated summary of its 25-year collection. The Center's current work includes interviews on tsunami in Hawaii and on Hawaiian Chinese restaurants.

Omaha Indian Music on American Memory from Library of Congress
memory.loc.gov/ammem/omh.html

Newly added to the American Memory historical collections is a major collection documenting the music of the Omaha Indian tribe. The collection includes 44 recordings made by Francis La Flesche and Alice Cunningham Fletcher between 1895 and 1897, as well as recordings made by staff of the American Folklife Center at the 1983 Omaha harvest celebration powwow and the 1985 Hethu'shka Society concert held at the Library of Congress. Also included with the collection are interviews with members of the Omaha tribe that provide background information about the songs performed, field notes and tape logs made by Center staff during the 1983 powwow, and photographs and related publicity materials from the various performances. Interviews with tribal elders, musicians, and singers provide contextual information and translations of the songs.

Chicago Historical Society and Museum
www.chicagohistory.org

This site has a wealth of information documenting Chicago's rich multicultural world. This contains Studs Terkel's recorded oral history archives, the oral history of the Polonia Project, and the Burr Tillstrom Collection and Archives.

Positive Exposure
www.positiveexposure.org

This organization was founded in 1997 by former fashion photographer Rick Guidotti and Diane McLean, MD, PhD, MPH, as an arts organization working with individuals living with genetic difference. Photography is used to document life histories.

Do History
dohistory.org

This site contains information on doing history, including oral history, interpreting diaries and journals, and analyzing mass media and film, as well as examples of projects. It was created by the Film Study Center at Harvard University and is hosted by the George Mason University Center for History and New Media.

Selected Oral History Centers, Archives, and Collections

- Baylor University Institute for Oral History
- British Library National Sound Advice
- California State University, Fullerton, Center for Oral and Public History Program
- California State University, Long Beach
- California State University, Monterey Bay, Oral History and Community Memory Institute and Archive
- Center for Documentary Studies at Duke University
- Chemical Heritage Foundation Oral History Program
- Columbia University Oral History Research Office
- George Mason University Oral History Projects
- Idaho Oral History Center
- Indiana University Oral History Research Center
- The Institute of Oral History, University of Texas, El Paso
- Kentucky Oral History Commission
- Living Legacies Historical Foundation
- Louisiana State University Oral History
- Maine Folklife Center
- Michigan Oral History Association
- Mississippi Oral History Project
- The National Archives
- National Library of Australia Oral History Collection
- Smithsonian Institution Oral History Collection
- St. Andrew's Oral History Project
- South Kingstown [Rhode Island] High School
- Southern Oral History Program, University of North Carolina
- United States Holocaust Memorial Museum
- University of Alaska Rasmuson Library Oral History Project
- University of California, Berkeley, Regional Oral History Office
- University of California, Los Angeles, Oral History Program
- University of Connecticut, Storrs, Center for Oral History
- University of Florida Libraries Oral History Collection
- University of Kentucky Oral History Program
- University of Nevada Oral History Program
- University of New Mexico Oral History
- University of North Carolina, Chapel Hill, Southern Oral History Program
- University of South Dakota
- University of Southern Mississippi Center for Oral Historical and Cultural Heritage

Note. May include digital archives or videotapes available upon request.

Selected Journals That Publish Oral Histories and Related Issues

Oral History Review

The *Oral History Review*, the official publication of the Oral History Association since 1973, explores the recording, transcribing, and preserving of conversations with people who have participated in important political, cultural, and economic social developments in modern times. Articles, book and film reviews, and bibliographies deal with the authentication of human experience and research findings in oral history. This journal considers a broad spectrum of different social groups, cultures, and countries through the use of interviews, songs, photos, diagrams, and storytelling. See further data on the OHA website for more detail.

American History Review

This is published online. It has been the official publication of the American Historical Association since 1895. It brings together multiple disciplines under the rubric of history. It is housed at Indiana University at Bloomington.

Narrative Inquiry

This journal publishes all genres of narrative inquiry. It is housed at Clark University Department of Psychology, Worcester, Massachusetts 01610-1477.

The Qualitative Report

Since 1990, *The Qualitative Report* (TQR) has been a leading publisher of qualitative work, including oral history reports and issues involving oral history. Since 2002 the publishers have received 678 original manuscripts from more than 50 countries. As posted on Google, TQR is the ninth largest ranked Web page in searches for qualitative research, and more than 1,500 sites worldwide have links to the TQR homepage. Currently there are around 3,000 readers and subscribers to TQR. All of this is free, and documents may be downloaded for free. Also, the site includes a weekly newsletter in electronic form, which anyone may subscribe to for free and that includes the latest articles published in the journal, conference news, and job postings. TQR spans all disciplines and welcomes interdisciplinary collaboration. Find the site as you Google *The Qualitative Report*.

Qualitative Inquiry

This is an interdisciplinary journal known for its creativity and lively discussions. All human sciences and topics are represented, such as in the areas of family studies, communication studies, oral history, medicine, education, social work, and many more.

New Media & Society

This journal has a wealth of articles and, of particular interest to the oral historian doing Internet inquiry, you will find articles on ethical beliefs and practices related to online research. The journal is a timely addition to the world library.

Sample Consent Form for Project Undergoing IRB Review

This study involves interviewing _____ about _____,
and is therefore research.

1. The purpose of this study is _____.
2. The study is expected to last from _____.
3. The number of people to be interviewed is _____.
4. The procedure of the research involves asking participants about their views on _____.
5. The interviews will be one hour each in length and each participant will be interviewed twice. The audiotapes will be protected in my home and will be kept for two years.
6. There are no foreseeable risks to the participants and they may leave the study at any time.
7. Possible benefits are educational, that is, to contribute to the body of knowledge about _____.
8. Members may choose to be completely anonymous and all names will be changed for reasons of confidentiality. This information will only be known to me and the chair of my dissertation committee.
9. For questions about the research, contact me _____ at _____.
10. Participation in this study is totally voluntary. Refusal to participate will not result in penalty or loss of benefits.
11. There is no cost to you to participate in the study.
12. The (name your university) Institutional Review Board (IRB) may be contacted at _____. This IRB may request to see my research records of the study.

I, _____,

(Please print your name above) agree to participate in this study with
_____. I realize this information will be used for educational purposes. I understand I may withdraw at any time. I understand the intent of this study.

Signed _____ Date _____

APPENDIX E

Basic Contract (Sample)

In consideration for the tape (or video) recording, editing, and preservation of my oral history interview (or oral memoir) by _____ (*name of archive, program or individual*) consisting of _____, I, _____ (*name of interviewee*), of _____ (*address*), _____ (*city*), _____ (*county*), _____ (*state and zip code*), herein relinquish and transfer to _____ my interview (or oral memoir) so that it may be made available to researchers and may be quoted from, published, or broadcast in any medium or form that the _____ (*archive, program or individual*) deem appropriate.

In making this contract I understand that I am conveying to _____ _____ (*archive, program, or individual*) all legal title and literary property rights which I have or may be deemed to have in my interview (or oral memoir) as well as my right, title, and interest in any copyright which may be secured under laws now or later in force and effect in the United States of America. My conveyance of copyright encompasses the exclusive rights of: reproduction, distribution, preparation or derivative works, public performance, public display as well as all renewals and extensions.

Signature of Interviewee _____

Signature of Agent/Representative _____

Date _____

Note. From the Oral History Association publication *Oral History and the Law*, by John A. Neuenschwander (2002, p. 80).

Federal Statement on Oral History

Oral History Excluded from IRB Review and Rationale

The U.S. Office for Human Research Protection (OHRP), part of the Department of Health and Human Services (HHS), working in conjunction with the American Historical Association and the Oral History Association, has determined that oral history interviewing projects in general **do not involve the type of research defined by HHS regulations and are therefore excluded from Institutional Review Board oversight.**

At the October 2003 meeting of the Oral History Association in Bethesda, Maryland, George Pospisil of the OHRP's Division of Education and Development, explained the OHRP decision regarding the application of the "Common Rule" (45 CFR part 46), which sets regulations governing research involving human subjects. These federal regulations define research as "a systematic investigation, including research development, testing and evaluation, designed to develop or contribute to generalizable knowledge." The type of research encompassed by the regulations involves standard questionnaires with a large sample of individuals who often remain anonymous, not the open-ended interviews with identifiable individuals who give their interviews with "informed consent" that characterizes oral history. Only those oral history projects that conform to the regulatory definition of research will now need to submit their research protocols for IRB review.

Following is the text of a policy statement that was developed by the Oral History Association and the American Historical Association in consultation with the Office of Human Research Protection. This policy applies to oral history that takes place within an institution that has filed a multiple project assurance with OHRP. As one of the seventeen federal agencies that have signed on to the Common Rule, the Department of Health and Human Services deals most directly with the type of clinical research that the federal regulations were originally intended to cover, and its concurrence with the policy statement should set the way for a uniform interpretation by other federal agencies. Oral historians should make this statement available to department chairs, directors of graduate study, deans, and other officers concerned with institutional compliance with federal regulations.

Donald A. Ritchie	Linda Shopes
Oral History Association	*American Historical Association*

Application of the Department of Health and Human Services Regulation for the Protection of Human Subjects at 45 CFR Part 46, Subpart A to Oral History Interviewing

Most oral history interviewing projects are not subject to the requirements of the Department of Health and Human Services (HHS) regulations for the protection of human subjects at 45 CFR part 46, subpart A, and can be excluded from institutional review board (IRB) oversight because they do not involve research as defined by the HHS regulations. HHS regulations at 45 CFR 46.102(D) define research as "a systematic investigation, including research development, testing and evaluation, designed to develop or contribute to generalizable knowledge." The Oral History Association defines oral history as "a method of gathering and preserving historical information through recorded interviews with participants in past events and ways of life."

It is primarily on the grounds that oral history interviews, in general, are not designed to contribute to "generalizable knowledge" that they are not subject to the requirements of the HHS regulations at 45 CFR part 46 and, therefore, can be excluded from IRB review. Although the HHS regulations do not define "generalizable knowledge," it is reasonable to assume that the term does not simply mean knowledge that lends itself to generalizations, which characterizes every form of scholarly inquiry and human communication. While historians reach for meaning that goes beyond the specific subject of their inquiry, unlike researchers in the biomedical and behavioral sciences they do not reach for generalizable principles of historical or social development, nor do they seek underlying principles or laws of nature that have predictive value and can be applied to other circumstances for the purpose of controlling outcomes. Historians explain a particular past; they do not create general explanations about all that has happened in the past, nor do they predict the future.

Moreover, oral history narrators are not anonymous individuals, selected as part of a random sample for the purposes of a survey. Nor are they asked to respond to a standard questionnaire administered to a broad swath of the population. Those interviewed are specific individuals selected because of their often unique relationship to the topic at hand. Open-ended questions are tailored to the experiences of the individual narrator. Although interviews are guided by professional protocols, the way any individual interview unfolds simply cannot be predicted. An interview gives a unique perspective on the topic at hand; a series of interviews offer up not similar "generalizable" information but a variety of particular perspectives on the topic.

For these reasons, then, oral history interviewing, in general, does not meet the regulatory definition of research as articulated in 45 CFR part 46. The Office for Human Research Protections concurs with this policy statement, and it is essential that such an interpretation be made available to the many IRBs currently grappling with issues of human subject research.

Statement on IRBs from the American Historical Association (Edited)

American Historical Association
THE PROFESSIONAL ASSOCIATION FOR ALL HISTORIANS

From the News column of the December 2004 **Perspectives**

Oral History and IRBs: Caution Urged as Rule Interpretations Vary Widely by Robert B. Townsend and Mériam Belli

Just as historians were beginning to think they could safely go back to oral history research without the possibly inhibiting oversight of institutional review boards (IRBs), some are finding progress blocked at the local level. While some universities have agreed that federal regulations were never intended to cover oral history research, many other institutional review boards are holding fast to rules that include oral history under human subject research—despite recent communications to the contrary from the concerned federal government office. As a result, oral historians in academia need to be aware of the policies and practices of IRBs at their home institution, both to ensure that they are in conformity with standing policies and to press for change where needed.

As regular *Perspectives* readers will remember, oral historians seemed to make significant progress on this front, when Michael Carome, the associate director for regulatory affairs at the federal Office for Human Research Protections (OHRP)—which is part of the Department of Health and Human Services—agreed that oral history interviewing activities "in general" fell outside the federal definition of research requiring scrutiny by IRBs. The AHA consequently issued an advisory statement suggesting that oral historians could now safely conduct interviews without IRB review (*www.historians.org/ Perspectives/Issues/2004/0403/0403new1.cfm*). The Oral History Association (OHA) also issued a similar statement. In a clarification issued on January 8, 2004, Carome *reaffirmed* the OHRP's concurrence with the policy statement as drafted by the AHA and the OHA (and modified according to suggestions made by the OHRP).

Despite this effort, a preliminary review of current institutional review policies in several universities, conducted by AHA staff and Zachary Schrag (an assistant professor at George Mason University), reveals that oversight of oral history projects remains a confusing patchwork of widely disparate poli-

Note. Retrieved from *www.historians.org/Perspectives/Issues/2004/0412/0412new4.cfm.*

cies and procedures. Some university policies, for instance at the University of Texas, seem to have adopted the position of the OHRP as stated in its communications (and contained in the AHA–OHA advisories) and have excluded, "in general," oral history interviews from IRB review (*www.utexas.edu/research/ rsc/humanresearch/special_topics/oral_history.php*).

In sharp contrast, a number of institutions are following a conservative line set by UCLA, which stipulates that "communication between OHRP and the oral history community does not change the HHS interpretation of the Federal regulations for the protection of human subjects nor does it change UCLA policy on such research" (*www.oprs.ucla.edu/human/NewsLetters/20031210. htm*). Still other institutions have remained silent on the issue, further compounding the general ambiguity.

"We are disturbed," observed Roy Rosenzweig, the AHA's vice president for research, "that some IRBs are not following the understanding the AHA worked out with the OHRP. But we feel that we owe it to our members to make them aware that some universities are insisting on IRB oversight of oral history."

The federal regulations on human subject research were designed for medical and psychological research that could inflict physical and mental harm on human beings, an aim reflected in the professional composition of most IRBs and the semantics of OHRP regulations. These regulations have been framed primarily to address research projects using interviews conducted with questionnaires and anonymous sources, not the type of open-ended, individualistic interviewing normally involved in oral history. Accordingly, the AHA and the OHA have argued that these regulations should not be applied across the board to the humanities and social sciences in general and oral history in particular.

Several legal scholars support this position. For example, C. Kristina Gunsalus—academic ethics expert, special counsel in the Office of University Counsel, and adjunct professor in the College of Law at the University of Illinois at Urbana-Champaign—asserts in a forthcoming article in *Ethics and Behavior* that oral history, like journalism and English, does not fall within the scope of IRB jurisdiction. She also insists that the related research currently subject to IRB regulations (surveys, informational interviews, etc.) would be best dealt with at the departmental level "rather than [left to] centralized review" (see *www.news.uiuc.edu/news/04/1011subjects.html*).

One repercussion of the present uncertainty has been a retreat to a cautionary stance by academic administrators and a certain degree of apprehension among historians doing oral history. By requesting IRB exclusion for oral history research, historians are simply affirming the distinct nature and purpose of oral history research (as compared to medical or even political science, despite interdisciplinary overlaps).

Despite the confusion on some campuses, the AHA continues to support the policy statement jointly elaborated with the OHA (*www.historians.org/press/2004_06_08_Council_IRBs.htm*) and agreed upon by the OHRP. However, given the legal uncertainties and complexities, the AHA cautions researchers doing oral interviews—especially graduate students for whom the stakes are particularly high—to carefully consult the institutional policy of their universities, as well as their department chairs, before undertaking fieldwork. This is imperative for all academic historians using oral interviews for their research, regardless of whether such interviews are the core of their work or only one source among many.

However, caution alone will not suffice. Historians—both as individual researchers and collectively as departments—must actively work within their universities to raise awareness about the potentially harmful effects of applying standards intended for a very different type of research to oral history.

—*Robert Townsend is AHA's assistant director for research and publications.*
—*Mériam Belli is a research associate for the Research Division of the AHA.*

List of Choreographers Used for Surnames of Participants

Mikhail Baryshnikov (b. 1948) is perhaps the most iconic dancer of our age. He was born in Riga, Latvia, danced for the Kirov Ballet in Leningrad, and defected to Toronto, Canada, in 1974. Since then he has achieved a level of greatness known only by a few other dancers and choreographers. His contributions to dance history are numerous. After freelancing as a lead dancer with various companies, he joined the New York City Ballet as a principal dancer and moved on to become artistic director of the American Ballet Theater. He has been an actor on stage, screen, and television and initiated numerous dance projects and partnerships with other choreographers, such as Twyla Tharp. He became a citizen of the United States in 1986. He cofounded the White Oak Dance Project with Mark Morris, which ran from 1990–2002. In 2004, he launched another project, the Baryshnikov Arts Center in New York City.

Agnes de Mille (1905–1993) was born in Harlem to a family well established in theater and film. Her uncle was film director and producer Cecil B. de Mille. She was passionate about dance and started studying ballet, then moved on to a more modern approach. She won fame for choreographing *Rodeo*, and then choreographed the dances for the film version of *Oklahoma*. She choreographed numerous Broadway shows. She founded her own dance company, the Heritage Dance Theater.

Martha Graham (1894–1991) revolutionized the dance world, changed how we view the dance world, and was known for her intense life and work. She is considered the most illustrious dancer and choreographer in terms of creating a paradigm shift in dance history. She is often considered the most influential and iconic innovator. She founded her dance company, which still performs worldwide to translate a new language of movement. She captured the rage, passion, and ecstasy of the human experience through concentration on the core center of the body as the strength to extend all other movement. She received numerous awards, accolades, and medals in her lifetime. Although she is considered the founder of modern dance, it can easily be said that she was so far ahead of her time that her dance statements are more postmodern in terms of expression. Graham was dancing and doing choreography until the end of her life.

Erick Hawkins (1909–1994) was born in Colorado. He moved east to study Greek history, civilization, and culture at Harvard, which greatly influenced his stylized modern dance. He worked in ballet and then modern dance with Martha Graham, whom he married in 1948. They were divorced in 1954. He founded his own dance company, and his choreography was influenced by Native American culture, Zen philosophy, and Greek classics. His famous book on dance is *The Body Is a Clear Place*.

Hanya Holm (1893–1992) was born in Germany. She gained fame and renown as a dancer, choreographer, and dance educator. She was influenced by and worked with Mary Wigman. She is often referred to as one of the major influences in modern dance. She was one of the founders of the dance program at Bennington College in the 1930s and taught in many colleges and universities in the United States before teaching at the Julliard School in New York City. She left letters, journals, and interviews for further study before her death in New York. Her technique emphasizing the use of space influenced many dancers who followed her, including Alwin Nikolai and Glen Tetley.

Doris Humphrey (1895–1958) was a contemporary of Martha Graham. Humphrey grew up in Chicago and is considered one of the pioneers of modern dance. Her emphasis on developing breathing techniques and interpreting movement continued the evolution of modern dance. The Doris Humphrey Society in Oak Park, Illinois, has a website and organization dedicated to her work and is notating her choreography.

Judith Jamison (b. 1943) was born in Philadelphia and began her dance career and training there. When she came to New York City she performed with the American Ballet Theater before joining the Alvin Ailey Dance Company. She became the artistic director and choreographer for the Alvin Ailey American Dance Theater shortly after Ailey's death. Ailey was her mentor. She also appeared on Broadway and did a PBS special on television on the creative process. She has received numerous awards for her choreography and continues to be active today.

Mark Morris (b. 1956) was born in Seattle, Washington, and grew up in an artistic family. Early on he moved to New York and founded his own company, the Mark Morris Dance Group. He is known for his creativity, ingenuity, and eclectic musical accompaniments to his choreography. He performed with numerous other well-known dancers and choreographers. He worked for 4 years with his company in Brussels, Belgium, and subsequently returned to New York. He then cofounded, with Mikhail Baryshnikov, the White Oak Dance Project to create new postmodern dances. He also choreographs for other companies, such as the San Francisco Ballet, the Metropolitan Opera, and the English National Opera. He is retired from performance.

Twyla Tharp (b. 1941) lived in Indiana and California before coming to New York. She is known for integrating ballet and modern dance, and her style is often referred to as "crossover" ballet. As with the other choreographers and dancers listed here she traveled the world with her dance company and performed as well on television and on Broadway. She has two Drama Desk awards, as well as a Tony Award. She collaborated with Mikhail Baryshnikov on many projects involving the fusion of ballet and modern dance.

Mary Wigman (1886–1973) was a German dance instructor and choreographer. Her protégé in the United States was Hanya Holm, and among Holm's students were the renowned Alwin Nikolais and Joanne Woodbury. In her choreography she often used non-Western music and percussion. She is considered the pioneer in modern dance in Germany.

Practicing the Techniques of Oral History

Strategies and Activities to Sharpen Your Writing Skills

1. To practice interviewing, find a member of your community to interview on the topic: What is your view of living here in _____? Practice with a digital voice recorder and practice uploading the interview on your thumb drive to a CD for transcription.

2. Complete a transcript of the interview. Read through the transcript carefully and see what themes emerge from the interview.

3. Practice journal writing every day for 1 week. Each day focus on writing in dialogue format with any one writer on oral history as method, on feminist oral history, or on issues of social justice, race, class, and gender in interviewing. For example, speak to the writers who influenced you, such as Dewey, Foucault, Giroux, Terkel, and so forth.

4. Write three pages on memories of your grandparents.

5. Write three pages on your earliest memory as a child.

6. Write three pages about your high school experience.

7. Write three pages about your college experiences.

8. Find a household item that annoys you and write three pages about why this item annoys you.

9. Select a photograph from your collection and write three pages on what that photograph means to you.

10. From a selected transcript, write three lines of poetry representing the meaning of that portion of the transcript. Use haiku, free verse, or rhyme, or all three.

Excerpt from an Oral History of a 9/11 Firefighter

From John Amato Interview. Date: January 2, 2002

A . . . At that point we were walking towards the building. We still didn't know it was a total collapse. As we get closer and closer, we notice that the smoke is clearing. We don't see the south tower. Now we're starting to talk to each other and started to actually worry what's in for us next. As we approached Chambers Street, kept walking, still no one had told us about the total collapse. We get down to about Barclay and Vesey Street, which is a block away from the overpass, the bridge overpass that goes across the West Side Highway. All you hear is a rumbling in the street. It sounded like an earthquake. When I was a younger kid, I was in an earthquake, and it felt like the same exact feeling. I looked, and I could see the antenna on the top of the roof coming straight down. We all turned and just threw our rollups down and started running as fast as we could. I took about five steps, I turned back to look behind me, and the debris was on my heels. Guys were just scrambling through the streets. Finally the debris overcame us, and you couldn't see anymore. It was like pitch-black, total darkness. I kind of ran into a building. I hit the building. One of the gentlemen working in the building I think I see was an engineer pulled me over towards the entrance. I went into the entrance. You couldn't see. It was dark as night. Finally a few minutes went by, about 4 or 5 minutes went by, it started clearing, and we started looking for members of Engine 68, as well as all the other engines that had driven down with us. We found everyone. We were told to stay at Chambers Street until further notice. That's about it. We stayed at Chambers Street. They didn't give us permission to go back in there, since we had already been involved with the collapse.

Q. So you stayed there for some period of time at Chambers, the staging area?

A. The staging area, yeah.

Q. And then from there you left? You took your rig back to 68 at some point?

A. Oh, yeah, I'd say about 11 P.M. that night. . . . Yeah, we stayed there the whole day.

Q. The whole day, and they never put you to work?

A. No. . . . They just didn't want anyone involved with the immediate collapse back in there. That was their idea. Since we were on paper as one of the companies, they didn't want us to go.

Q. Is everybody from 68 okay?

A. Yeah.

Note. Retrieved from oral histories from September 11 compiled by NY firefighters (*http:// graphics8.nytimes.com/packages/pdf/nyregion/20050812_WTC-GRAPHICS/9110421.PDF*).

APPENDIX K

Excerpt from an Oral History of Hurricane Katrina Survivors

This page contains featured oral histories. These oral histories cover the time interval between the first announcements that a hurricane was coming to the time the respondents were interviewed, in January–March 2006. The site will follow respondents over time in additional interviews. As these updates become available, links will be created so that listeners can follow the story of a particular respondent across multiple interviews.

000382: This respondent was staying with friends at the time of the hurricane. She decided not to evacuate. She feels fortunate because, in her opinion, she was not too badly affected by the storm. At the time of the interview, she explained that one of her biggest frustrations is dealing with her insurance company. She states that "it will never be normal here again."

400793: A woman explains that during the storm she lost family members, and is continuing to have problems with her insurance company. However, she finds that she is much better off than many others and is assisting victims of the hurricane.

404506: Initially, this respondent's family was reluctant to evacuate, but along with several family members, he decided to go to his daughter's home in Nashville. After several days without any news about his home, a friend called to let him know that his home had been severely damaged. When he finally was able to go home, he found that his house was still standing. He discusses why he is grateful for the assistance that the Red Cross provided. He also explains his frustrations with his insurance company and FEMA [Federal Emergency Management Agency]. He has been staying in a FEMA trailer, and is still not sure if he and his family are going to stay where they are or move elsewhere. He still finds himself lucky when compared to what others went through.

404675: This respondent evacuated the Sunday before the storm arrived. He discusses the difficulties of evacuating, such as traffic, not being able to find a hotel room, and having a pet pass away. Several days after the hurricane, he was told that he could go back home, but due to the lack of availability of gas, he could not make the trip at that time. When he did make it home, he found a lot of damage, but now feels that his life is pretty much "back to normal." He and his family are planning on moving from Louisiana.

Note. Retrieved from *www.hurricanekatrina.med.harvard.edu/oralhistories.php*. These are audio files, so this appendix is a summary of some of the responses. To listen to the audio files, go to the website and click on a file.

Example of a Nonparticipant Observation Assignment to Develop Observation Skills

Where: Restaurant, coffee shop, shopping mall, zoo, place of worship, museum, health club, funeral parlor, skating rink, or any public setting.

Why: To observe a complex public setting. There should be natural public access to the setting and multiple viewing opportunities for you. This exercise is to sharpen your observation skills.

How: Nonparticipant observation. Go to this social setting more than once to get a sense of the complexity and to maximize what you learn. Go at least TWO times (three times preferred) at different times of the day. If you wish to return at any other time, of course, feel free to do so. Take notes. Make a floor plan or take photos. If possible, try to connect your observation to a history of the place you are observing. Try to find a social justice issue.

1. The setting: Look around you and describe the entire physical space. Draw a floor plan or take a photo, if permitted.

2. The people: Look around you and describe the people in this setting. Focus on one or two of the people. What are they doing in that social space?

3. The action: What are the relationships between people and/or groups? Try to discover something about the people in the setting.

4. Describe the groups and any common characteristics, for example, age, gender, dress code, speech, activity, and so on, or focus on one person in your viewing area to describe in detail. For example, a waitress, a caretaker, a salesperson, and so on, depending on your setting.

5. If you had all the time in the world to do a study here, what three things would you look for upon returning to the setting?

6. Be sure to give a title to your report that captures your observational study.

7. Be sure to use references from our texts this term or any other appropriate texts.

In your self-reflection include (1) How has this performance activity challenged you?; (2) What difficulties did you encounter in the field setting?; (3) What would you do differently if you were to return?; (4) What did you learn about yourself as a researcher?

APPENDIX M

A Sample Rubric Assessing Writing

Name _____ Date _____

Course: Qualitative Methods   First Assignment _____

Strengths in Your Work

_____ Work handed in on time

_____ Ideas presented clearly and with appropriate examples, title accurately reflects content

_____ Creativity and imagination evident

_____ Connected texts from the class to your writing

_____ Appropriate conclusions, summary, and recommendations

_____ Evidence of serious reflection

_____ Use of appropriate research examples

_____ Other: meets page requirement/goal

_____ Attached field notes/transcripts or other documents as needed

_____ Responded to questions, including serious extended reflection on self-evaluation, difficulties in the field, and lessons learned as a researcher

Comments on strengths:

Areas for Improvement

_____ Need to show evidence of serious, layered, reflection on the topic/conclusions/introductions

_____ Need to develop stronger summary, conclusions, and recommendations

_____ Need to indicate your rationale for selection of site/topic

_____ Need to show evidence that you read the class texts and to connect ideas from at least one if not all three required texts authors in your work

_____ Need to work on punctuation, grammar, and paragraph development

_____ Need to focus your work, especially in _____

_____ Need to read and follow directions

_____ Need to focus on graduate writing and/or on narrative writing

Comments on areas for improvement:

Class Discussions/Presentation

_____ High Pass

_____ Pass

_____ Low Pass

_____ Did not verbally contribute

You have earned the following grade on your first project:

Interview Project Assignment

This assignment is due on final class date.

Reminder: This project cannot be handed in any later. No exceptions.

Project: Interview one person twice, so that you have the experience of going back for an interview. Interviews should be at least one hour in length each. The topic of the interview is: **WHAT DOES YOUR WORK MEAN TO YOU?** Select an educator or other professional to interview about what work means to that person. The first interview should have some basic grand-tour questions like the following:

INTERVIEW PROTOCOL A—FIRST INTERVIEW

1. What does your work mean to you?
2. Talk about a typical day at work. What does it look like?
3. Tell me what you like about your job.
4. Tell me what you dislike about your job.
5. Where do you see yourself in 5–10 years?

You create the questions for **INTERVIEW PROTOCOL B. You create the questions based on what you found in the first interview and to get to the goal of the interview.**

This should take at least an hour, but no longer than 90 minutes per interview. Aim for each interview to take an hour of time. Be sure to take field notes so you can probe into areas of this first interview during the second interview. Be sure to tape all this. Be sure to get informed consent. Use either of the sample consent forms that appear in the book "Stretching" Exercises for Qualitative Researchers (Janesick, 2004).

Due on last class night: A paper/report of 15–25 pages, in which you do at least the following:

1. Describe in detail why you selected this person.
2. Provide a list of all the questions asked in each interview and label them. Interview Protocol A, Interview Protocol B.

3. Summarize the responses from both interviews in some meaningful way, with precise quotations from the interview.

4. Pull out at least **THREE THEMES** from the interviews.

5. Tell the story of what this person's life work means to this person.

6. Include the signed consent form.

7. Discuss any ethical issues that may have come up.

8. A sample of three pages of your best transcript from the tape.

9. **Include a page or more of your own reflections** on your skills as an interviewer and as a researcher and what you learned from this project; be sure to mention any difficulties that came up and what you will change the next time you conduct an interview.

10. Be sure to use references from our texts this term.

11. Be sure to create a title that captures your themes.

Remember that this is a narrative research paradigm, so you should write this in narrative form as if you were telling this person's story. The story is about the person's life work.

Example of a Qualitative Research Methods Syllabus

Course Syllabus for EDF 7478-901 Qualitative Research Methods in Education

Tuesdays, 15-week course, 4 credits

Instructor: Valerie J. Janesick, PhD, Professor
 Office: 158 J
 Phone: (813) 974-1274
 E-mail: *vjanesic@tempest.coedu.usf.edu*

The Theoretical Frame of the College:
The College of Education CAREs

The College of Education is dedicated to the ideals of Collaboration, Academic Excellence, Research, and Equity/Diversity. These are key tenets in the conceptual framework of the College of Education. Competence in these ideals will provide candidates in educator preparation programs with skills, knowledge, and dispositions to be successful in the schools of today and tomorrow. For more information on the conceptual framework, visit *www.coedu.usf.edu/ main/qualityassurance/ncate_visit_info_materials.html.*

How This Framework Connects to the Current Class

In this course, learners will conduct research with the spirit of excellence in technique, in collaboration with participants, and with an awareness of finding the stories and voices of those usually on the margins of the dominant social group.

Note. This is my syllabus; I focus on narrative approaches such as oral history, life history, portraiture, and some archival approaches.

Themes

Under the look of fatigue, the attack of the migraine and the sigh
There is always another story, there is more than meets the eye.
        —W. H. AUDEN, from the poem "At Last the Secret Is Out"

Artistic form is congruent with dynamic forms of our . . . life; works of
art are projections of "felt life" as Henry James called it, into spatial, tem-
poral, and poetic structures. They are images of feeling that formulate it
for our conception.

                                                —SUSANNE LANGER

Course Description

This course deepens the understanding of qualitative research methods,
design, data collection, analysis, and interpretation. It builds on prior qualitative course work whenever possible. Participants will analyze and interpret
observation and interview data, as well as learn techniques to analyze documents, archival techniques, and multimethods integration, as needed and if
appropriate. Use of digital cameras and video recorders will be a central technique studied this semester. Ethical issues in field work and the role of the
researcher will be key topics for discussion and writing. **Individuals ready to
begin proposal writing for the dissertation are encouraged to complete Chapter 1 and/or 3 of the proposal.**

Goals

In this course you will be expected to:

- Complete all readings and in-class assignments.
- Master and **deepen library research and archival skills** and the use of
  BLACKBOARD.
- Deepen your practice of interviewing and observation skills.
- Identify your theoretical framework, such as phenomenology, critical
  theory, interpretive interactionism, chaos theory, existentialism, con-
  structivism, feminism, aesthetics, dramaturgy, etc.
- Identify which of the qualitative case approaches suits you, such as oral
  history, ethnography, case studies, autoethnography, life history, visual
  ethnography, portraiture, narrative inquiry, photo voice, etc.

- Continue practice in writing analytical vignettes based on field work and practice writing poetry from interview data.

- Discuss the artistic components of telling someone's story and deepen your understanding of artistic approaches in the qualitative genre.

- Discuss in small groups and the group as a whole problems related to field work, including ethical issues that arise in research.

- Continue the study of major writers in the field and learn how to read research articles as a reflective, critical, active agent.

- Understand the knowledge base underlying various approaches to research.

- Understand which questions are suited to qualitative research techniques.

- Practice using digital tape recorders and video recorders and digital film techniques as data collection tools and integrating Web-based resources into your work.

- Demonstrate advanced proficiency in use of Web-based resources and use of documentary evidence.

- Read, write, discuss, and reflect upon key issues in qualitative research methods, including issues of race, class, and gender, issues of practice such as locating oneself ideologically, purposeful sampling, ethical issues in field work.

CHECK BLACKBOARD DAILY.

Instructional Methods

Small-group discussion and group work, computer lab and library work, projects in and out of the classroom. Some guest speakers to be announced, some lecture/demonstration/ discussion, minilectures as needed. Documentary film and follow-up discussion; new techniques for transcribing interviews.

Equipment Needed

It is helpful to have a **digital voice recorder for interviews**. Although a mini-cassette works, most transcribers prefer the digital voice recorder with the thumb drive insert, such as the Olympus 1100 or higher. Or any MP3 player or iPod with appropriate attachments. The cost of a digital recorder is anywhere from $50 up to $150. Many students buy their equipment at any major discount store. Many transcription services prefer digital technology for ease and immediacy of use.

It is optional, but a digital **camera or a combo digital camera and video recorder** is also quite helpful. The most user friendly and affordable is the FLIP IT 60-Minute Ultra Camcorder with built-in USB. This records up to 60 minutes of an interview (for those who decide to do video interviews). The cost is around $150. This type of unit also plugs into the TV monitor so you can see your interview or observation at any time in class or at home. Note: Eight megapixels or above is highly recommended.

Optional Foot Pedal System for Those Doing Their Own Transcripts: Olympus makes a device for about $120. And you need to weigh that against the going rate for transcriptions in the open market. Currently, the cost for transcribing a 1-hour interview from a digital voice recorder is around $110. If you use a minicassette recorder, the cost is higher.

Professional Transcription Services: Check transcription rates at the top transcription center in the United States, which is in Los Angeles, at *www.productiontranscripts.com*; also check *www.castingwords.com*. Local transcription services are also available. These will be announced in class.

Required Reading

All class members will read these texts in common.

Creswell, J. (2007). *Qualitative inquiry and research design: Choosing among five approaches* (2nd ed.). Thousand Oaks, CA: Sage.

Kvale, S. (1996). *InterViews: An introduction to qualitative research interviewing.* Thousand Oaks, CA: Sage.

Janesick, V. J. (2004). *"Stretching" exercises for qualitative researchers* (2nd ed.). Thousand Oaks, CA: Sage.

Cole, A., & Knowles, G. (2001). *Lives in context: The art of life history research.* Lanham, MD: Alta Mira Press.

If doing a qualitative dissertation, this text is highly recommended:

Piantinida, M., & Gorman, N. (1999). *The qualitative dissertation.* Thousand Oaks, CA: Corwin.

Select one of these optional texts, which are completed qualitative studies or notes on method, for your reading and future use.

Gawande, A. (2007). *Better: A surgeon's notes on performance*. New York: Metropolitan Books.

Goldberg, N. (2005). *Writing down the bones*. Boston: Shambhala Press.

Reinharz, S. (1992). *Feminist research methods in social research*. New York: Oxford University Press.

Mazzei, L. (2007). *Inhabited silence in qualitative research: Putting poststructural theory to work*. New York: Peter Lang.

Kingsolver, B. (2006). *Animal, vegetable, miracle: A year of food life*. New York: HarperCollins.

Try to select a text in the area in which you will concentrate: oral history, life history, narrative research, ethnography, narrative inquiry, portraiture, etc. All texts should be current. Use the 10-year rule. Remember, you will be building a collection of texts for your methods section of the dissertation. You must build your library in the content area and methods area.

Electronic and Other Resources for Qualitative Researchers, Including Journals, Websites, Listservs, Software, Etc.

All class members go to *www.aera.net/Default.aspx?id=777* for a list of relevant sites. Also check blogging sites for qualitative researchers.

There are key journals in hard text and online journals that focus on qualitative inquiry. There are numerous Web resources and transcription services. See pages 124–142 in Janesick (2004).

Check out the e-journal *The Qualitative Report* online: *www.nova.edu/ssss/QR/index.html*

Assignments

There will be two major written assignments for all members:

1. Analysis and interpretation of interview transcripts based on last semester's interview project for those who completed an interview study, including 10 pages of actual transcription, 20–30 pages. This is 30% of your grade. Due at the fifth class.

This is for those who have taken at least one qualitative class and have completed at least two interview transcripts. Or, if you have already done this activity, you will write a complete description of your theoretical frame for your qualitative research project, including a review of all relevant literature.

Members who join us for the first time will do an observation assignment as described below.

Each class member must pass, at the proficiency level, the following tasks IN CLASS:

a. Participant observation exercises, including field notes, thick description, preliminary informed hunches, and what-would-you-do-next text for:
- Observation of a still-life scene.
- Observation of a social setting.
- Observation of a person.

b. Interview, transcription, and preliminary data analysis of same for:
- Interview of a person you know.
- Interview of a stranger.

Transcriptions of at least 30 minutes of taped interview with field notes, preliminary categories for follow-up, and set of informed hunches. Remember that 1 hour of taped interview data is 21 typed pages. You may use your interview project to fulfill this requirement.

c. Practice with digital photography as needed.
d. Document review as needed.

2. Mini-Proposal—Sample sections of your dissertation proposal. Should include any two sections of the following: Introduction and Purpose Statement, Theoretical Framework for the Study, Methodology, Categories of Related Literature. This is 40% of your grade.

Those who are not at this point yet will conduct either another interview assignment or a document analysis assignment.

New members who join this class and have not had a qualitative course before this one will do an interview project.

There will be three in-class writing assignments with Pass/Fail grading. Each class member must pass, at the proficiency level, the following tasks:

1. Journal writing session on description of the role of the researchers.
2. Journal writing session on the ethical issues inherent in the project.
3. Writing session on the following:
   a. Statement of the problem and purpose of the study.
   b. Exploratory questions that guide the study.
   c. Theoretical frame of the study.
   d. Methodology selected and techniques described.

   e. Developing a model of what occurred in the study.

   f. Practice at selecting exact quotations from transcripts.

NOTE: TO MAKE UP A MISSED CLASS, PROVIDE A 5-PAGE PAPER ON THE TOPICS FOR THE READING AND YOUR REFLECTION ON THEM FOR THAT CLASS. DUE THE FOLLOWING CLASS.

REMEMBER TO CHECK BLACKBOARD DAILY.

Assignment 1: Nonparticipant Observation Assignment: To develop observation skills. Due the fifth week of class.

Assignment 2: Interview Project Assignment. Due the final class evening.

GRADING

1. Students must inform the instructor before the due date if an assignment will not be ready on time. Students who are absent must find someone to take notes and pick up any class handouts for them. Students may have one free pass for missing one class.

2. Students must inform the instructor before class when and if they will be late or absent from any class.

3. If a student is late with a written assignment, a penalty will be included in the grading process of a flat 5% off your given grade. Also, if you do not hand in an assignment, you will be assigned the default grade of B– for the entire course.

Each project is worth:
a. Observation project or transcripts assignment   30%
b. Interview project or literature review or description of your   40%
   theoretical frame
c. In-class participation and attendance, contributions to discussion   20%
d. Technology proficiency (takes place in library at tech session, date   10%
   TBD in the first half of the semester)

   4. Grading is based on the following scale:

100–95	A
94–90	A–
89–86	B+
85–80	B
79–75	C

Note: The grade of C– or lower is unacceptable in graduate studies. Please be sure to get a copy of the University's Graduate Catalogue, which spells out the policy. You must complete all requirements in this class. There are no Incomplete grades given in this class. You will be graded upon what you complete.

Standard rules of etiquette apply in class.

Topics and Schedule: Subject to Change

[There follows the list of dates and assignments.]

The class is planned in three major sections: intro to approaches, sharpening and performance practice exercises, and sharing work with the entire group. Discussions cover ethical issues, skills as an observer, interviewer, and writer, learning new digital techniques, presenting documentary evidence, and working with documents and photographs.

Plagiarism

Copying someone else's work is a very serious offense and can bring about a student's removal from the program and the university. You plagiarize when, **intentionally or not**, you use someone else's words or ideas without giving them credit. Quotation marks should be used whenever you are using the exact words of another author. Square brackets and ellipses should be used to indicate any words that are deleted from the original material. Summarizing a passage from another source or rearranging the order of a sentence or sentences is paraphrasing. Every time you paraphrase the work of another author, you should give credit to the author by citing. If you are using someone else's ideas, you must give them credit as early as possible in your text. In this course, if you are found guilty of plagiarism, you may receive an F (Failure) in this course and be dropped from the program. USF has strict rules on academic dishonesty. Check the Graduate School Policies and Procedures Manual immediately.

Please do not make me put your work through the plagiarism checkpoints.

An Excerpt of a Transcript (Edited) from an Interview with Jane A. de Mille

Q: Okay, since I haven't seen you in a while, can you talk a little bit about what you're doing right now, the role you have, a little bit about the people you work with in the district, and just your typical day?

A: Sure. Sure. Well, I'm starting my 5th year now as assistant superintendent in an elementary district of about 1,600 kids, south suburbs. Which, in the 4 years I've been there, is going through a demographic shift; it was probably the last White, predominantly White suburb and is now becoming pretty integrated. You know, most of the south suburbs are either Hispanic or Black. We seem to be becoming a good balance. So the last 4 years I've dealt with . . . the areas of responsibility are really curriculum technology, ELL [English language learners], bilinguals, reading improvement, everything but special ed, and the budget, basically, comes under my jurisdiction. Right now, special ed because the special ed director's on maternity leave. So the big umbrella really is helping people deal with change: the changing demographics, the changing expectations for students, the changing regulatory aspects of No Child Left Behind. So it was a very staid community. People were there for 30 years, and they retired. You know, it was their first job, it was their last job. And I came at the end of a 3-year wave of retirements. So now there are a handful of veteran teachers, a good chunk of mid-career people (meaning maybe 10 to 15 years), and lots of "newbies." So. . . . And a lot of focus on curriculum, creating district-wide curriculum. When I got there it was building based. It could be grade-level based. We had maybe seven different math curricula being used in the elementary schools feeding into one junior high. Things like that. So creating a sense of community has probably been my biggest focus.

Q: Now tell me a little bit about your superintendent: male, female, does the person have a doctorate like you have?

A: Sure. He. . . . This is his 8th year. He is. . . . This is his first, and I'm going to venture it's going to be his only superintendency. He is a Renaissance person. He started life as a social worker and worked in mental health, worked in a mental health school. Decided he wanted to go into law, got a law

---

Note. Jane was questioned on her role as a female assistant superintendent. Notice the social justice themes that emerge.

degree. And absolutely hated the practice of law. So he does have. . . . He's got a JD. And then went back into the social work aspect and went through and got an administrative background. So he's been a social worker, a school principal, county-wide director of special ed and now a superintendent. He likes the job a lot but he is. . . . He could retire right now and has contemplated retiring and then going to work. . . . He lives near a neighboring state so he could retire in Illinois and go work in a neighboring state and. . . . In another year he'll have four girls in college and he keeps thinking, hmm, maybe I should take that 75% pension and get another real job. So. . . .

Q: Talk a little bit about what you studied in your bachelor's, master's, how long were you a teacher, were you a principal, all those things.

A: My initial bachelor's is in special ed with visually impaired and elementary ed. And at that time that wasn't an option, you had to do both, because most visually impaired kids are in regular classes, so, so I have both of those degrees. Never actually taught straight-vision [visually impaired] kids, because by the time I was getting out of school most straight-vision kids didn't go to collective programs, they were itinerant. So I did do itinerant work with a few straight-vision kids, but a lot of kids with [multiple] needs. And left teaching for a year because I was tired of working two jobs. I was also a shift manager for McDonald's. And I worked as a manager for McDonald's, where I could only have one job, which was nice. But I really did miss teaching and the state. . . . Illinois opened a residential program for students who were deaf/blind in the north part of the state, in Glen Ellyn. And I applied and went to work there. And it was a very cool program. It's a small school, maybe . . . probably at its largest could house maybe 30 to 35 kids. Extended day program, took two shifts of teachers. Kids went to school from 8:00 in the morning to 8:00 at night, so 8:00 in the morning until 3:00 was one shift of teachers, 3:00 until like 9:30 was the second shift of teachers. So that kids got education across all domains in the community. Eventually in public schools, through a program that the state had launched, the kids left home and were in local public schools, we had classrooms in local public schools. Left the classroom there and became a . . . the consultant that worked with other teachers and parents and did staff development and parental training for the state through that program. And then, on a dare, basically, left that position to support a student who was deaf/blind in a [multiple] needs classroom in Skokie. And from there was mentored by the all-female administrative team there, and went into administration there. So . . . then moved onto Naperville, where I got to open a new school. . . . And then just went to interview for this position because I was interested in learning about the multi-age school that they had, because I had interviewed a teacher from this district when they were moving farther away, and decided to take the position, and then saw an ad for the assistant superintendent position. So this was my 26th, 27th, one of those, one of the upper 20 years of education. Yeah. [pause]

Q: Think about yesterday and today, not necessarily as typical days, but what does your day look like from the minute you get up, what is it. . . . Tell me all the things you deal with and we'll go from there.

A: Well, it's been a typical day so that's. . . . And that's something I've been thinking about. There isn't . . . there are typical days and they're boring. The typical days are the days when you're sitting and working on paperwork for the state and working on budgets and trying to analyze test scores to make them meaningful to the teachers and to the . . . and whatever. So those are the typical boring days. This is our second week of school, so there's no typical beginning of the school year. Now I'm spending more time supporting teachers, right now new staff. Right now I'm doing . . . pulling on my special ed background. I have a little guy who is in one of our self-contained classrooms, but he's struggling with the transition coming back to school, and mornings aren't good for him, and he's got a new teacher. And the principal in that school is on maternity leave. And the principal who is filling in was a little panicked. And so we met and talked about strategies for this little guy that, no, you know in first grade he's not ready for therapeutic day school. He's not hurt anybody. Everything's fine. It will be okay. We have a controversy going on right now related to curriculum materials that have been selected for students' optional use, optional reading. So we've been laughing and . . . on one hand . . . and cringing on the other because we're responding to one parent's concern.

We have only heard from one parent who has a concern about a book that was on the summer reading list. Kids take home a list of six or seven books that are optional. The kids give a synopsis of the book at school. They talk about them. And if you don't like any of those books, you can read any other book in the whole wide world to choose from. And this one is as much young adult literature as it is controversial themes because it gives us the opportunity to support kids as they worry about these things and . . .

Q: Can you tell the name of the book and . . .

A: It's *Fat Kid Rules the World* by Kale Going. And the themes really are friendship, not giving up, perseverance. A student in there contemplates suicide. He's had a very tough time. His mom's died from cancer. His dad's an alcoholic. He's in an abusive home situation. And he is befriended by a homeless teen who is a gifted guitarist who asks this kid to join his band and play the drums. And it basically is about acceptance, and you know it's a great story of redemption. It's a wonderful story. And the parent that objects is objecting based on the proliferation of the *f* word. And it is in there and it . . . kids are in Brooklyn. And interestingly enough, but it's not really spoken out loud. It's in this kid's thoughts. That she's objecting to the normal sexual fantasies of teenagers. He's describing a person and saying no, not this one, not the one with the large breasts, you know, the other one . . . physical features. So, you know, things like that. This parent has, you know, not accepted the fact that her child was not required to read the book and. . . . She did not ask for the book to be banned from the library. I think she just asked for it to come off the summer reading list. However, that has snowballed to some right-wing websites . . . Concerned Women for America, the Illinois Family Network. I don't know which all . . . Save Libraries.org. And we have been getting interesting e-mails from basically all over the country and Canada.

Q: What would be an interesting e-mail?

A: Oh, some that are saying. . . . One was, you know, "If I knew where Osama Bin Laden was, I would turn him in, but first I would tell him where your school was so that he could bomb it. Hopefully when there was no children . . . on the weekends when no children were present." You know, "You're responsible for the moral degradation of children and the increase in rapes and murders and school shootings because children have read . . . because we have forced children to read this book." Personally, me as a woman, I'm not fit to lead, even though, Lord knows how that's connected. I'm not sure. We were joking that a bunch of us are Catholic so we were all damned already anyway, so it didn't matter, so you know. It's been real very. . . . The Board's been very supportive. They . . . you know, they listened to an hour and 10 minutes of different people expressing their viewpoints. Some people had heard it on the radio, a Board member from a distant suburb came to express her concerns. Somebody from our Library Board came. The phone call from one of the mayors in one of the towns that we serve. But the Board was supportive and said that, you know, no, this was not required reading, that the teachers did inform students that, you know. We did make an error in not informing parents that they, you know, that they might want to be alerted to this fact. And so we are looking at our selection policy and how we let parents know where they might want to . . . if they want to follow up. But in all of this time since our last Board meeting, and since this started in mid-August, we have only heard from that one parent.

Q: Have you been threatened, or has anybody?

A: I have not personally been threatened. The junior high principal has been threatened. You know, "When someone comes and murders your family, it'll be because of how you taught them." Rather interesting. No one from the immediate community. . . . No other parents in the community. . . . There's an article in today's paper, we had a prepared statement to share with people who called anticipating . . . and this is the daily paper. This is not like the local "Podunk" paper. We had one parent phone call with a question or concern. And we did end up sending a note home today, you know, saying that, you know, we didn't believe that the threat was really credible but that we did have, you know, that there was a police presence.

. . . It was on the book list for incoming eighth graders, so that would be 13- and 14-year-olds. They talk about these things. And some statistic that I had recently come across said three to five . . . three out of five teenagers contemplate suicide at one point. So, um . . . yeah, it's kind of important to maybe say, yeah, there's a place to talk about this. It was . . . it's probably towards the young end of the age spectrum that the book might be appropriate for. And we did have a parent come and talk in support of the book. Her child had read it during seventh grade. He's a very capable student. And as a parent she also read the book and thought it was a perfect avenue to discuss some of these difficult situations, which some of our students live in. You know we don't. . . . Not everyone lives in a two-parent home where they go to church every Sunday and their other social, emotional, and physical needs are met. Literature is one way to talk about kids who are sitting next to you or are on the other side of the country who don't have those same experiences. This student obviously and this parent who was able to sit and talk with her child about these things who a year later recalled that the themes were, you know. . . . Didn't recall the swearing, didn't recall the sexual fantasies, recalled the overarching themes. We have students that haven't read an entire book probably since they were in second grade who were talking about how fabulous the book was. Kids whose lives unfortunately probably mirror the protagonist's life.

So as a result of this, as we were pulling up reviews, just off of Amazon, to give parents a synopsis of the book, we did look at one of the books that was being offered to our honor seventh graders. And we did decide to take it off the list. Because we thought it might be a little too graphic. It dealt with sexuality issues and homosexuality.

And it is a big topic for kids. And it is an issue that we think needs to be explored. And it was an optional book. It's for a lit circle about self-acceptance. But that maybe there's another . . . a better option out there. Because just because the kids can read at that level it doesn't mean that maturity wise they're able to.

Q: Now thank you for sharing the e-mail that was sent to you, but for the purposes of the transcript here, can you describe . . . can you describe the contents briefly of that e-mail that you received? This is from, again, only one parent over this one book.

A: Well, this is a person. I don't even know who it is. He equated the ability of a woman to be president and whether or not he should vote for a woman as president with my role as an assistant superintendent in this school district and the analogy of someone who comes upon a boat that has a little bit of water in the bottom and drills a hole in the boat to let the water out and continues to drill additional holes to let more water out as of course more water's rushing in, and some man miraculously comes and says no, no, maybe we should stop drilling holes and plug the holes instead and saves the day. And who should we vote for, the man that plugs the holes or the woman who has drilled the holes? And in his warped sense of the world he also sent. . . . Prior to my e-mail my superintendent received an e-mail with just a shortened version of that analogy but accusing him of being a hole driller as well. But I obviously am not . . . or women in general are not fit to be president because we obviously must be the hole drillers. There might be some warped men who also are stupid enough to drill holes with us. But we as a gender probably are sucking them into it. So, that would be atypical. . . . If I get an e-mail from a parent it's generally related to a curricular concern or a testing question.

Q: So and let's say you get this e-mail then. How do you deal with it? What strategies do you use or what is that like?

A: Well, I'm not deleting it, only because I'm saving it just for posterity. Other than that we get a lot of good laughs out of it, we shared it around the office. And you go on with your day. Exactly. It will be good for a laugh at many times in the future.

I spend more time in my office at my desk now filling out forms for pittances from the government than I've ever done before. Much more accountable for every dime that the federal government gives us. I spend time working with teachers. I spend time working with principals. Tried to create a leadership study group really among the administrative team. We've done some book chats. I think this year we're going to do articles. There's a group in Illinois called Midwest Principals Association that offers some really relevant high-quality peer offerings for administrators. And then every year they have what they call marquee speakers. And this year the speakers are Andy Hargraves, Doug Reeves, Heidi Hayes-Jacobs, and Pedro Neguerro. So I think what we're going . . . I'm going . . . we're going to do this year, and I'm kind of the person responsible for planning that, is do . . . I'm going to do some articles by those people prior to those. So we do some of those leadership support activities as professional development.

About the authors, about what their passions are, what their perspectives are. And I'm hoping that we will all go as a group to those presentations because those are all people that, even if you could only see them for one day, can make a big impact on your . . . on your learning. Right now I'm also doing a lot of data analysis and working with the principals and the Building Leadership Teams about student achievement, what we know about what kids. . . . How kids are testing. What do we know about what's happening in the classrooms and what do we have to do differently.

Q: Could you talk a little bit about School Board meetings you have to attend, how often, how many, and so on?

A: The School Board is my friend. I attend all School Board meetings. Our Board officially meets only once a month. We do not have regular standing committees, which is great. Right now, though, we have been going through contract negotiations, and we're going through strategic planning. We've just completed a strategic plan, and so the Board is formalizing action plans for that. I do go to and report at every Board meeting. I participate in all closed sessions, so in that way there's no differentiation between the superintendent and myself.

He does the Board packet. I flesh it out, basically, you know, with all the information that goes to it. So . . . yeah, I'm a regular.

Q: Then, you know, you mentioned that you . . . you're doing data analysis on achievement and so on. How has No Child Left Behind affected you? Can you speak a little bit about that?

A: No, no, no. It's affected me, actually, primarily in positive ways. While I know that it's ludicrous and I'm looking, you know, that all children are going to achieve, what it has enabled me to do is given me the other way to say sorry, we have to look at this, data that we needed to be looking at anyway. Why are our. . . . You know, why are certain groups of children not achieving? Looking at our curriculum, not looking at schools per se or grade levels per se. . . . Well, no, actually looking at grade levels across the district and saying, why are we not moving forward? Why are our kids not meeting the state standards? You know, is there something wrong with the state standards? What, you know, let's talk about what's the expectations. Are they not realistic? So it's been a great cause for dialogue. It's helped me move forward the need to support ELL students across the curriculum, to support special ed kids across the curriculum. Where in the past and the old guard was, if you were an ELL student, if you were a special ed student, well, you were in my class, but I didn't have to take any responsibility for you.

It's easy for me to push you off on somebody else, even though that "somebody" might have been two ELL teachers across four schools with 200 students. I didn't have to take responsibility for you. So for me it's been a wonderful lever to. . . .

Q: Talk about . . . let's talk about this ELL, English language learners?

A: Right. I mean—to a degree, yes, and in other ways, no. I think Illinois has done a very nice job of having high expectations for ELL students. The perfect case, I had a meeting today with all our ELL teachers, and we're testing new kids and kindergarteners coming in. And we're part of a multistate consortium and really took a lead in developing with Wisconsin, with the Center for Linguistics out of University of Wisconsin, developing the test that we use for English language acquisition and whatever. And being a blue-collar suburb, middle to low-middle income, we have students who are dual-language students who qualify for services based on a new statewide standard that, quite frankly, are above our typical kindergarten class. And that that odd sense of trying to explain to a teacher why the student must get some kind of ELL services even though they are a leader in the classroom. They have more literacy skills. They have more background knowledge because many of our students. . . . They can be Spanish, Arabic. Spanish and Arabic are our two predominant languages. Polish, Romanian are also big. Polish comes and goes. We have another big Polish push. Our Arabic is not. . . . Varies. We've had a big Jordanian population. Now we've had a big Yemeni group. So and that varies and then that varies on their . . . the parents' literacy background. The Hispanic population is predominantly Mexican. I would say those are our biggest groups.

So, yeah. Big Yemeni group recently. We've had big Polish groups. When I came 4 years ago Polish was our biggest second language.

So we get many more immigrants first . . . this is their first place. So before it was, they came to the city, then they migrated to a first-string suburb, which we are. And then they would. . . .

Yeah. And more spread across our three schools. It used to be we had a school that had more Arabic, a school that had more Spanish, and then a school that didn't have as much. Now all three of our elementary schools are probably equal . . . not equally Hispanic and Arabic but have a good solid group of both sets of parents.

Q: So now let's talk about, if you will, some of the decisions that you made that you're really proud of and what went into that. What, as an assistant superintendent, are you really, really happy about, so that some day you can say "I accomplished this." Or talk a little bit about what you really think worked and what goes into that? What do you draw upon?

A: I have been very fortunate to work in organizations who . . . where at some level, not always at every level that you would like, but at some level always focus on what's right for kids. That when it comes down to A or B, what's chosen is what's best for kids. And that started back in Skokie, which was a very mixed community where I supported that young girl who was deaf/blind, where I became . . . that was my administrative background. Where we had an entire women administrative team who all had . . . we used to joke that people would probably call us "the coven." And we all had different strengths. We were an . . . you want to talk about a high-performing team. Our superintendent had been trained with Larry Lizotte. She had come out of Michigan out of his initial Essential School stuff. She worked at . . . She was an assistant superintendent in Michigan. And we truly . . .

everyone brought different strengths to the team. And we would have meetings where we just had knock-down, drag-outs over philosophy and whatever. But you want to talk about a place where at least 50% of the kids were trilingual. We had no tax base whatsoever. Kids . . . you know, parents were either Northwestern professors or working three jobs because they were political refugees from, you know, Nigeria or Algiers or wherever, where kids were achieving at high, high levels. You know, predominant. . . . To be religiously mixed there was a big deal. You'd go to a bar mitzvah where . . . I'd go to a kid's bar mitzvah where there would be, you know, Catholic kids and Hindu kids and Jewish kids and Muslim kids.

It was like the U.N. It was in Skokie, yeah. It is. It was very much U.N. And we were in the center of Skokie. We didn't have much. We didn't have industry. We didn't have Old Orchard Mall. We had a very limited residential tax base, so very different . . . Skokie has six elementary districts, so it has very different financial supports. So, you know, big Indian population, whatever. So it was very interesting, very interesting. Because it was a predominantly Jewish board? Yes, a Jewish board. They were able to say, you know, our students are no longer predominantly Jewish, our staff is not predominantly Jewish, it is important that we take care of all the kids. So we will no longer take the holidays off, that we will certainly allow staff to take those holidays off and students to take those holidays off. We were on NBC News. . . .

Yeah, we were on NBC News when the Board voted to no longer take the high holidays off. As far as I know, in the northern suburbs it may still be the only district that does not take the high holidays off.

So that focused . . . I mean that focused on kids. And then I got the opportunity to open a brand-new school in Indian Prairie, which was probably at the time the fastest growing school district in the country. Went from a consolidated unit district, which in Illinois there's unit districts and elementary and secondary districts. The small . . . it was a rural consolidated district that began to grow in the west end of Naperville. And was really, even when I came aboard, and I opened the 16th or 17th elementary school in the district, still very much operated as a small district. The assistant superintendent for elementary, really about that time, when I was opening the school, came to the realization that he did not know every elementary teacher anymore. Never came to grips with it, but did you know. . . . They did not have systems in place to operate a district of 20 and now they have 30 schools, you know, covering 45 square miles and 25,000 to 30,000 students. They were still operating on the I know that you . . . I know you. . . . You know, I know you, Jane Smith, and I'm going to open a new school and I need you, Jane Smith, because you have this knowledge base to go help with this new school. And I know you, Jane Johnson, and I know that this building needs some relief from you, Jane Johnson, and you're not really damaging the kids but you're not really doing a whole lot of good, so you also are going to go help that school. I was that last group of people who were actually handpicked by the assistant superintendent for who was coming from the school that was serving my students, who was being chosen to come and join me, some good and some bad. And then I hired the rest of the people so. . . . It was awesome! And it was very difficult to decide to leave there. It was fabulous. I really got to create a. . . . That was probably the proudest thing of my career, a fabulous, fabulous school community that was truly. . . . We. . . . Most kids walked to school. They'd always taken a bus. I had huge parent involvement. I had fabulous teachers. I had a very diverse school, which was uncommon in the district. There was either. . . . It was either, you know, the haves or the have nots, there was very few that were both. Very . . . some . . . very wealthy schools, country club communities. And then some that had a lot of apartments and Section 8 housing. I really had a blend of both. When they opened a new subdivision in my attendance area of what would be move-up houses, many of my parents sold their starter homes and moved to the move-up houses, because they didn't want to leave [their current school]. Very family oriented. We had things that brought us together. We unfortunately had a teacher die of breast cancer, so we supported kids as they went through that. We had a real strong PTA who. . . . And me, coming from a multicultural background, I got to influence them and say, you know, when we have an event on a Friday night and everybody here is White and we don't have any of our Hispanic families or our Black families or our Indian families, why is that? Can you . . . you know, who can you talk to in your neighborhood to find out what's the problems? You know, how do we make sure everyone's included? My very last all-PTA event that I was at was our end-of-the-year picnic, which we had every year. Unfortunately, the weather was bad, so it was inside. And we had some kind of reenactment, some kind of. . . .

It was some kind of medieval reenactment thing going on. And so there was guys with swords and all this other stuff, some people that the PTA brought in. And I just. . . . This picture of this guy who was this reenactment guy with this armor on and this long flowing hair and showing them this shield and his sword and these three dads sitting around. And one dad was Indian and one dad was Black and one dad was White. And that truly was what my school looked like, 5 years after it opened, when I left. It was truly a neighborhood community that came together. We . . . unfortunately, had . . . went through the loss of several parents from cancer and some other things, and ALS, and a community that so totally came together to support one another. . . . Unfortunately, the person who came after me was there for 1 year and almost destroyed it in one fell swoop. . . .

Q: You said . . . you used the words "servant leadership," and you serve those kids in the district.

A: I laugh. My biggest job is the question asker. In a very nonjudgmental open way. And it's. . . . Last year we started a science committee. It's the third curriculum committee that we're working on since I've been there. And some new people on there, people who hadn't been on a committee before. And I'm like, "No, no, no. You're misunderstanding. I have no answers." And science is the best one for me to say, "Listen, I know nothing about science. I can ask questions, and you guys need to guide me so I know what to bring to the committee to look at." You know. "I am the facilitator of . . . I'm the gatherer of the information. I will find resources whether they're print or people, whatever. But I'm the person that's just going to ask you the questions." I think that's the easiest way to start letting people see that they have a voice. When we started a math curriculum adoption, it was not a good curriculum work. It was really a textbook adoption. We didn't do any curriculum writing. We were in a crisis mode. And I was like, how can I facilitate this so that everyone knows that they have input? And we literally released every classroom teacher to come to a meeting during the day where we get . . . it was an hour and a half or whatever by grade level where one of the principals facilitated a grade level and I facilitated a grade level, to ask them what they liked about what they had going in math right now. What did they want to make sure that we replicated? What were their concerns? What were they . . . they say their needs? They were blown away. They were like, I can't believe you're asking me. You know. People are always given an opportunity for a voice. I never have a committee where I'd say X number of people can be on the committee. It's always open to whoever wants to come. So I don't care if I have everybody from one grade level at one building. I do go seeking more people if there's not representa-tion. But it's still. . . . Because people still aren't trusting of that their voice is really the voice that's being heard. You know they don't really. . . . We went through that . . . with that math adoption. We did piloting. We did train. . . . You know we did some piloting. We got together, and all I did was ask questions when it came down to deciding what math materials to adopt. And they just kept saying, well, what do you want? I said, "It doesn't matter what I want. I'm not in the classroom. I think you've selected three things that are all really good. I don't think we'll go wrong with any of them." "Well, which one costs more?" "It doesn't matter what they cost." We were in a financial pinch at the time. It doesn't matter. We're going . . . "I've committed to buy everything that you need to implement this program. And I mean everything. Anything that you see on the list of all, the wish list from the publisher, whatever you want, I'll buy." You know. They did not know how to have those conversations. We had adopted a new curriculum,

6 to 8. And the sixth-grade teachers also then kind of sat in the middle. And they did then move along like. . . . Well, this is my concern about this one, because I know now where kids need to be to move forward. I think this might be good here. I can understand why you like this. I'm not sure that's not going to get us where we want to go. Nobody knows to this point. . . . Everyone thinks and they talk about, oh, it was such a good thing that you brought this curriculum. They didn't pick what I wanted. They picked something else.

It's wonderful. It's worked fabulously. They've done a great job. We did staff development for the whole trimester before the next year started. Everyone was totally trained. We had days' worth of training. It was a totally big, big shift for them. And it's been fabulous. It was the first time everybody in the district could have a conversation about something because they had a shared experience. They had a shared expectation in the classroom. That had never happened before.

. . . And probably because good, bad or indifferent, what's good for kids always drives. . . . When push comes to shove, what's good for kids has always driven the decisions. You know, careerwise, I'm going. . . . This is really odd to say this, but careerwise, taking this position was probably the dumbest thing I ever could have done. The south suburbs are viewed negatively in Chicago. I took a lateral pay move, and I'm probably making less money now than I would be if I was still principal where I had been before. But I believed in the vision that the superintendent had for excellence, that being average wasn't good enough. And that was the vision for the district, was being average was okay, you know, that being average was all right. Then excellence is what we should expect for our students. I've made a big difference in how people view children of color and ethnically diverse kids and the expectations they have for kids, not in every classroom but in lots of classrooms. So while personally and for my career it was probably a stupid move, in the lives of kids, and that was . . . the purpose was to expand my circle of influence, it's been a good move. Might I have made a similar move, had I stayed where I was? Yeah, maybe I would've. You know, that crystal ball, the person who. . . . You know, the curriculum person left the district I was in. Subsequently, that same year, they filled it with an interim for a year, and then somebody who . . . a colleague of mine who I respect whose background was not significantly different than mine took the curriculum position in that very large unit district. Might that have been me? Sure. It might have been. But, you know, I was an irritant there, just like I was an irritant here. I was like, I was a change agent.

APPENDIX Q

Digital Equipment for the Oral Historian

The models and prices I am listing here are subject to change as new products are developed, but this list provides guidelines as to the type of features that are offered as of the publication of this book.

Digital Voice Recorders (price range from $39 to $199)

1. **Olympus VN-6000.** This recorder has 600 hours of recording time and a long-life battery.
2. **Olympus WS 400S DNS.** This recorder has about 272 hours of recording time.
3. **Olympus VN 5000.** This recorder has 330 hours of recording time, voice activation, and USB connectivity.
4. **Sony ICD–BX700.** This recorder has a 1GB flash memory, holds 280 hours of recording time, and is voice activated.
5. **Livescribe Pulse Smartpen.** This pen is a voice recorder and comes in 1GB and 2GB sizes. 1GB captures 100 hours of recorded audio.

Digital Video and/or Camcorder

1. **Flip Camera.** This camera is lightweight, has video and audio high performance, and can record up to 2 hours of interview data at a time. It has Flip-Share software, connections to any digital TV, and multiple accessories. This is known as the Flip Mono HD or Flip ultra HD. Price range is $120 and up, depending on accessories.
2. **IPOD models.** IPOD models with video accessories may record audio and/or video. Price range is $200 and up, depending on digital storage.

References

Alexander, T. M. (1987). *John Dewey's theory of art, experience, and nature.* Albany, NY: SUNY Press.

Altheide, D., Coyle, M., DeVriese, K., & Schneider, C. (2008). Emergent qualitative document analysis. In S. N. Hesse-Biber & P. Leavy (Eds.), *Handbook of emergent methods* (pp. 127–154). New York: Guilford Press.

Blee, K. (1993). Evidence, empathy, and ethics: Lessons from oral histories of the Klan. *Journal of American History, 80*(2), 596–606.

Clark, E. (1999). Getting at the truth in oral history. *Social Research and Social Change, 6,* 1–18.

Cohen, D. J., & Rosenzweig, R. (2006). *Digital history: A guide to gathering, preserving, and presenting the past on the web.* Philadelphia, PA: University of Pennsylvania Press.

Creswell, J. W. (2007). *Qualitative inquiry and research design: Choosing among five approaches* (2nd ed.). Thousand Oaks, CA: Sage.

Csikszentmihalyi, M. (1996). *Creativity: Flow and the psychology of discovery and invention.* New York: Harper Perennial.

De Mille, A. (1992). *Martha: The life and work of Martha Graham.* New York: Vintage Books.

Denzin, N. (2001). *Interpretive interactionism.* Thousand Oaks, CA: Sage.

Dewey, J. (1925). *Experience and nature.* New York: Dover.

Dewey, J. (1934). *Art as experience.* New York: Penguin.

Freire, P. (2007). *Pedagogy of the oppressed.* New York: Continuum.

Frisch, M. (1990). *A shared authority: Essays on the craft and meaning of oral and public history.* Albany: State University of New York Press.

Frisch, M. (2008). Three dimensions and more: Oral history beyond the paradoxes of method. In S. N. Hesse-Biber & P. Leavy (Eds.), *Handbook of emergent methods* (pp. 221–238). New York: Guilford Press.

Giroux, H. (2006). *America on the edge.* New York: Palgrave Macmillan.

Goldberg, N. (2005). *Writing down the bones: Freeing the writer within.* Boston: Shambhala.

Hawkins, E. (1992). *The body is a clear place and other statements on dance.* Pennington, NJ: Dance Horizons.

Hesse-Biber, S. N., & Leavy, P. L. (2007). *Feminist research practice: A primer.* Thousand Oaks, CA: Sage.

Hesse-Biber, S. N., & Leavy, P. (Eds.). (2008). *Handbook of emergent methods.* New York: Guilford Press.

Janesick, V. J. (1999). Using a journal as reflection in action in the classroom. In D. Weil (Ed.), *Perspectives in critical thinking: Theory and practice in education* (pp. 173–195). New York: Peter Lang.

Janesick, V. J. (2000). The choreography of qualitative research design: Minuets, improvisations, and crystallization. In N. K. Denzin & Y. S. Lincoln (Eds.), *Handbook of qualitative research* (2nd ed., pp. 379–399).

Janesick, V. J. (2004). *"Stretching" exercises for qualitative researchers* (2nd ed.). Thousand Oaks, CA: Sage.

Janesick, V. J. (2007a, March). Oral history as a social justice project: Issues for the qualitative researcher. *Qualitative Report, 12*(1), 111–121.

Janesick, V. J. (2007b). Reflections on the violence of high-stakes testing and the soothing nature of critical pedagogy. In P. McLaren & J. Kincheloe (Eds.), *Critical pedagogy: Where are we now?* (pp. 239–248). New York: Peter Lang.

Kincheloe, J. (2007). Critical pedagogy in the twenty-first century: Evolution for survival. In P. McLaren & J. Kincheloe (Eds.), *Critical pedagogy: Where are we now?* (pp. 9–42). New York: Peter Lang.

Kvale, S. (1996). *InterViews: An introduction to qualitative research interviewing.* Thousand Oaks, CA: Sage.

Kvale, S., & Brinkmann, S. (2009). *InterViews: Learning the craft of qualitative research interviewing* (2nd ed.). Thousand Oaks, CA: Sage.

Lee, S. (n.d.). Interview. Retrieved from: *www.hbo.com/docs/programs/whentheleveesbroke/interview.html.*

Leistyna, P. (2007). Neoliberal non-sense. In P. McLaren & J. Kincheloe (Eds.), *Critical pedagogy: Where are we now?* (pp. 97–123). New York: Peter Lang.

Lincoln, Y., & Tierney, W. (2004). Qualitative research and institutional review boards. *Qualitative Inquiry, 10*(2), 219–234.

Lofland, J., Snow, D. A., Anderson, L., & Lofland, L. H. (2006). *Analyzing social settings: A guide to qualitative observation and analysis* (4th ed.). Belmont, CA: Wadsworth.

Mallon, T. (1995). *A book of one's own: People and their diaries.* Saint Paul, MN: Hungry Mind Press.

McLaren, P., & Kincheloe, J. L. (2007). *Critical pedagogy: Where are we now?* New York: Peter Lang.

Neuenschwander, J. (2002). *Oral history and the law.* Carlisle, PA: Oral History Association.

Perks, R., & Thomson, A. (Eds.). (2006). *The oral history reader* (2nd ed.). New York: Routledge.

Pink, D. (2006). *A whole new mind: Why right-brainers will rule the future.* New York: Berkley.

Progoff, I. (1992). *At a journal workshop: Writing to access the power of the unconscious and evoke creative ability.* Los Angeles, CA: Tarcher.

Reinharz, S. (1992). *Feminist methods in social research.* New York: Oxford University Press.

Ritchie, D. (2003). *Doing oral history.* New York: Oxford University Press.

Rose, G. (2007). *Visual methodologies: An introduction to the interpretation of visual materials* (2nd ed.). Thousand Oaks, CA: Sage.

Rubin, H. J., & Rubin, I. S. (2005). *Qualitative interviewing: The art of hearing data* (2nd ed.). Thousand Oaks, CA: Sage.

Schön, D. (1983). *The reflective practitioner: How professionals think in action.* London: Temple Smith.

Shea, C. (2000). Don't talk to the humans: The crackdown on social science research. *Lingua Franca, 5*(1), 27–34.

Shostak, M. (1981). *Nisa: The life and words of a !Kung woman.* New York: Random House.

Tharp, T. (2003). *The creative habit: Learn it and use it for life.* New York: Simon & Schuster.

Thompson, P. (1988). *The voice of the past: Oral history* (2nd ed.). New York: Oxford University Press.

Tutu, D. (1999). *No future without forgiveness.* New York: Doubleday.

Yow, V. (1994). *Recording oral history: A practical guide for social scientists.* Thousand Oaks, CA: Sage.

Yow, V. (2005). *Recording oral history: A guide for the humanities and social sciences* (2nd ed.). Lanham, MD: Alta Mira Press.

Index

ABOUT THE AUTHOR

Valerie J. Janesick, PhD, is Professor of Educational Leadership and Policy Studies at the University of South Florida, Tampa, where she teaches classes in qualitative research methods, curriculum theory and inquiry, foundations of curriculum, ethics, and educational leadership. Her text *Stretching Exercises for Qualitative Researchers, Second Edition* includes ways to integrate the arts in qualitative research projects, and she is currently working on the third edition, which will include the technology connections and the use of poetry to represent interview data. Dr. Janesick's writings have been published in *Curriculum Inquiry, Qualitative Inquiry, Anthropology and Education Quarterly*, and other major journals. Her chapters in the first and second editions of *Handbook of Qualitative Research* use dance and the arts as a metaphor for understanding research, and her chapter in *Handbook of the Arts in Qualitative Inquiry: Perspectives, Methodologies, Examples, and Issues* addresses John Dewey and the arts and education. She is completing oral history interviews of female school superintendents as part of a larger project on women leaders and is currently taking classes in yoga and meditation. Her most prized possession is her British Library Reader's Card, in particular for her work on an archival project on John Dewey's letters to international educators and their subsequent influence.